G000021494

BRACHYTHERAPY: TYPES, DOSING AND SIDE EFFECTS

CANCER ETIOLOGY, DIAGNOSIS AND TREATMENTS

Additional books in this series can be found on Nova's website under the Series tab.

Additional E-books in this series can be found on Nova's website under the E-books tab.
'

CANCER ETIOLOGY, DIAGNOSIS AND TREATMENTS

BRACHYTHERAPY: TYPES, DOSING AND SIDE EFFECTS

LEONI M. FISCHER
EDITOR

\\

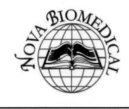

Nova Science Publishers, Inc.
New York

Library of Congress Cataloging-in-Publication Data

Brachytherapy : types, dosing, and side effects / editor, Leoni M. Fischer.
p. ; cm.
Includes bibliographical references and index.
ISBN 978-1-61728-750-3 (hardcover)
1. Radioisotope brachytherapy. I. Fischer, Leoni M.
[DNLM: 1. Brachytherapy--methods. 2. Brachytherapy--adverse effects. WN 250.5.B7 B7965 2010]
RC271.R27B73 2010
615.8'424--dc22
                      2010022568

Published by Nova Science Publishers, Inc. † New York

Contents

Preface

Brachytherapy, also known as internal radiotherapy, is a form of radiotherapy where a radiation source is placed inside or next to the area requiring treatment. Brachytherapy is commonly used as an effective treatment for cervical, prostate, breast, and skin cancer and can also be used to treat tumours in many other body sites. Brachytherapy can be used alone or in combination with other therapies such as surgery and chemotherapy. This book presents current research from around the globe in the study of brachytherapy including High Dose Rate (HDR) Intracavitary Brachytherapy for cervical, breast and prostate cancer, as well as nanobrachytherapy and Brachytherapy for soft tissue sarcomas.

Chapter 1 - The increasingly routine use of prostate surface antigen (PSA)-based screening has led to the diagnosis of more patients with organ-confined prostate cancer. These localized cancers are routinely treated with radical prostatectomy, external beam radiation therapy or prostate brachytherapy. Prostate brachytherapy is an appealing treatment for reasons including patient convenience, a favorable toxicity profile and cost-effectiveness. Consequently, the utilization of brachytherapy is increasing, both in the United States and around the world. Although there are no randomized trials comparing the various treatment modalities, and long-term efficacy data are somewhat limited, the available evidence suggests that prostate brachytherapy achieves favorable results in lower risk patients that rivals those achieved with radical prostatectomy and external beam radiation therapy in terms of local control, prevention of biochemical relapse, and prevention of prostate cancer specific and overall mortality. As improved risk stratification and imaging modalities increase the accuracy with which patients with organ-confined disease can be identified, these results can be expected to improve. In addition to better patient selection, ensuring the proper dose is delivered also impacts the efficacy of treatment. Improved techniques such as three-dimensional intra-operative planning can increase the likelihood that a sufficient and homogenous dose is delivered to the entire prostate including all suspicious or known lesions identified by clinical exam, imaging and prostate biopsy. In part due to these diagnostic and technical advancements, prostate brachytherapy may be an effective treatment for localized intermediate-risk disease, both as monotherapy and in combination with external beam radiation therapy.

Chapter 2 - Purpose: To evaluate the outcomes, toxicities and dose-volume histogram (DVH) parameters of high-dose-rate interstitial brachytherapy (HDR-ISBT) in the management of primary and recurrent gynaecologic malignancies.

Materials and Methods: Between 2001 and 2009, 38 patients with gynaecologic cancer were treated at L'Hotel-Dieu de Quebec with Ir-192 remote afterloading HDR-ISBT, using a Syed-Neblett template for implant technique and inverse planning simulated annealing (IPSA) algorithm for dosimetry optimization. The median HDR-ISBT dose delivered was 30Gy (range: 18–35), given in 4–6 Gy/fraction. All patients received pelvic external beam radiation therapy (EBRT). Four patients with vaginal recurrence (R) also had previous intracavitary brachytherapy (ICBT). Toxicities were assessed according to CTCAE v3.0. Total equivalent dose in 2-Gy fractions (EQD2) was calculated, combining HDR-ISBT and EBRT contributions. Results were compared with published data.

Results: Of the 38 patients reviewed, 30 were treated for primary malignancies (PM) of the vagina (n=15), cervix (n=9), vulva (n=2) or Bartholin's gland (n=4) and 8 had recurrent gynaecologic cancer. FIGO stage distribution for PM was: I (n=2), II (n=12), III (n=13), IV (n=3). Median age was 57. Median follow-up was 20.6 months (range: 1-92). Complete response rate (CR) was 82% for PM versus 75% for R. Local control (LC) for PM and R was 86.7 vs 37.5% at 2 years and 81.3 vs. 37.5% at 5 years (p=0.007). 5-year overall survival was 78.9 vs 14.3% (p<0.001). DVH parameters for target volume showed a median V100 of 97.5% and EQD2 D90 and D100 of 89Gy10 and 69Gy10. For OAR, median dose to 2cc (D2cc) was 80.1Gy3 for rectum and 76.9Gy3 for bladder. These DVH values appear to be at least equivalent to those published for MRI guided ICBT following the GEC-ESTRO recommendations, except for our rectal D2cc that was higher. The median D0.1cc for urethra was 79.7Gy3. Twelve patients experienced grade 3-4 late toxicities (gastrointestinal and genitourinary) but only two of them were still suffering from grade 3-4 toxicity at last follow-up.

Conclusion: The use of HDR-ISBT offers good long-term LC, especially in PM, at a cost of possible transitory severe late toxicities. This therapeutic option should be considered for PM that cannot be optimally treated with ICBT and for isolated R. DVH parameters of OARs recommended by the Gyn GEC-ESTRO and urethral D0.1cc or D10 should be reported. Further investigations are needed to define dose-volume constraints in HDR-ISBT.

Chapter 3 - High-dose-rate (HDR) intracavitary brachytherapy (ICBT) is widely applied for patients with cervical cancer. The advantages of HDR-ICBT are time and resource conservation, outpatient service, convenience, and optimal cost-effectiveness. Meta-analysis shows similar local control and complications in comparison with low dose rate ICBT. The rectum is the most common organ at risk (OAR) in the reports about HDR-ICBT. The International Commission on Radiation Units and Measurements (ICRU) 38 report defined reference points for dosimetry. The rectal complications are related not only to cumulative ICRU doses to the rectum, but also to external parametrial doses (PMD). For diminishing biologically effective dose (BED) of the rectum, rectal balloon inflation, small fraction size of point A, or intensity modulated radiation therapy (IMRT) may be beneficial to patients with potentially high rectal doses. Correlations between dosimetry and complications of the urinary bladder and sigmoid colon are controversial due to organ movement. CT/MRI-based treatment planning is suggested for more accurate dosimetry because doses of ICRU reference points are typically underestimated using orthogonal radiography-based dosimetry. To improve local control rate, MRI-guided brachytherapy is preferred for better target delineation and dose coverage. The unsolved issues of HDR-ICBT are weighting relative to external beam radiation therapy, dose rate effect, impact of concurrent chemotherapy, optimal dose-fraction, interfractional dose variation, brachytherapy devices, dosimetry using 3D planning, and reference points/volume for OAR. This chapter presents a comprehensive literature review and discussion.

Chapter 4 - In the present paper a therapeutic option for the treatment of Basal Cell Carcinoma (BCC) and Squamous Cell Carcinoma (SCC) is described. It basically consists in a superficial high dose brachytherapy, characterized by the use of a ready-to-use kit, in which a radioactive beta-emitting isotope, incorporated in a specially formulated inert, synthetic resin, is applied on the surface of BCC and SCC tumours. When the product is applied on the lesion, a beta emitter brachytherapy irradiation is performed, strictly limited to the area and depth affected by the tumour invasion. The electrons from high energy (> 1MeV) beta emitters isotopes deposit more than 90 % of the dose to the first two mm of the skin, which is the depth usually interested from tumour invasion, but spare the deeper tissues from irradiation. The therapy has been used in a large variety of BCC and SCC: tumours of very large sizes, relapsing or recurrent forms, multifocal lesions, without restriction of site, dimension, clinical or histological type, patients clinical situation, with exclusion of the lynphonode metastatic forms. More than 1200 lesions on 370 patients, with histologically, dermoscopically, or clinically confirmed diagnosis of BCC and SCC, have been treated. After a follow up of 12 - 78 months, a complete response was obtained in 98% of the treated lesions, in 89 % of the lesions after a single application, while in 11% of the patients two or three treatments were performed. A clear advantage of the proposed treatment respect to the surgery is especially evident for all the tumours located in difficult sites, on which surgery would be difficult (nose, ears, eyelids, etc.). The technique should be, in our opinion, the first choice treatment in all those patients with a high number of lesions, or with tumour relapses, in those with tumours located in particular sites, where surgery would produce functional mutilations (penis, vulva, eyelids etc.) and, finally, in older, infirm, or otherwise inoperable ones.

Chapter 5 - Breast cancer treatment has changed substantially in the past several decades. Initially, all women were treatment with mastectomy. However, this is a major and often a very difficult surgery for the patient, both physically and emotionally. Several studies were published that demonstrated acceptable local control and equivalent survival when mastectomy was compared with whole breast irradiation (WBI) following the surgical removal of the tumor[1,2]. This shifted the treatment paradigm as the new standard of care became 5 – 6 weeks of radiation delivered to the whole breast. Although a survival benefit for WBI has not been demonstrated in prospective, randomized trials, a metaanalysis suggests that there may be a small benefit for women less than 60 years of age [3].

Chapter 6 - The use of balloon brachytherapy devices for High Dose Rate (HDR) partial breast irradiation is well established. Alternatively, balloon applicators can be used for HDR brachytherapy treatment of gynecological malignancies. This includes treatment for (1) post operative endometrial cancer and (2) inoperable endometrial cancer. Here, we describe the clinical and dosimetric methodology for these two treatment sites.

Balloon devices were used as applicators for vaginal vault irradiation for patients treated post-operatively and for treatment of the uterus for those with inoperable endometrial cancer. Patients were treated with a Varian iX Ir-192 high dose rate brachytherapy source. Three dimensional treatment planning was done with BrachyVision 8.2 and was based on CT scans acquired for each treatment fraction.

For irradiation of the vaginal vault, the use of a balloon applicator reduces the frequency of air gaps between the vaginal mucosa and the applicator as compared to a standard segmented cylinder applicator. It provides excellent radiation dose coverage of the target area with acceptable doses to the bladder and the rectum. For treatment of the uterine serosa, the dose distribution is similar to that obtained through the use of Simon-Heyman capsules while maintaining the ease of a single-entry applicator. It also provides a more reproducible treatment because the volume of the balloon is easily duplicated from fraction to fraction. The insertion and removal of the applicator in both treatment sites is well tolerated.

The use of balloon applicators in gynecological sites is a clinically feasible and safe method of patient treatment. Balloon applicators offer the simplicity of a single-entry, single channel tool. The applicator itself is patient specific based on the fill volume of the balloon and can be the same from fraction to fraction, or can adapt if the patient anatomy changes. The dose distributions obtained are similar to conventional treatment devices. Other treatment sites may also benefit from the use of a balloon applicator.

Chapter 7 - Brachytherapy is an important cancer therapy modality. The common cancers for which this kind of therapy is useful include skin cancer, prostate cancer, cervical cancer,etc. This kind of treatment has been used in Thailand for a long time, and many reports on this cancer treatment have been done there. In this specific article, the author summarizes the important reports on brachytherapy in Thailand. Special focus is placed on types, dosing and side effects.

Chapter 8 - Nanomedicine has become the new emerging medical science. It can be applied to many branches of medicine. Application of nanomedicineto cancer therapy can be seen, and nanobrachytherapy is the newest approach for brachytherapy. This article will briefly discuss this new approach of brachytherapy.

Chapter 9 - Limb-sparing surgery and adjuvant radiation have replaced amputation as the mainstay treatment for patients with soft tissue sarcoma (STS) of the extremity, since adjuvant radiotherapy has been shown to improve local control and disease-specific mortality. Additional brachytherapy, interstitial tumor bed irradiation, following conservative surgery represents a means of enhancing the therapeutic ratio, as biological and dosimetric advantage over external beam radiotherapy (EBRT).

Success in the management of STS is often limited by the extension of lesions to neurovascular structures. In an effort to preserve limbs, conservative surgery with adjuvant high-dose-rate (HDR) brachytherapy has been reported, whereas little is known about the tolerance of peripheral nerves to brachytherapy. The purpose of this study was to determine the oncological outcome in patients with STS treated with adjuvant HDR brachytherapy and to evaluate the efficacy and radiation neurotoxicity of HDR brachytherapy in patients with STS in contact with neurovascular bundles.

Between 1995 and 2000, 28 patients with 29 STS of the extremity and superficial trunk were treated in our institute with limb salvage surgery followed by fractionated HDR brachytherapy. Seven of the 28 cases involved the neurovascular bundle. Afterloading catheters placed within the tumor bed directly upon the preserved neurovascular structures were postoperatively loaded with Iridium-192 with a total dose of 50 Gy. To further investigate the subclinical nerve damage by HDR brachytherapy, motor nerve conduction velocity studies were carried out in 3 patients.

There was one local recurrence and 8 lung metastases. Eighteen patients survived and continued to be disease-free. One patient died of heart problems. With a median follow-up period of 34 months, the 5-year actuarial overall survival and disease-free survival rates were 68.1 and 51.9%, respectively. Complications included 4 wound complications, 2 nerve damage, and one bone fracture. But there was no practical and electrophysiological finding of neurotoxicity due to HDR brachytherapy.

This study demonstrated that conservative surgery combined with adjuvant HDR brachytherapy is the treatment of choice for patients with STS to avoid amputation or major limb function loss. Several large clinical studies have established the efficacy of conventional low-dose-rate brachytherapy as an adjuvant therapy for STS. The use of HDR is considered to be an attractive alternative, because this technique allows treatment to be given in minutes instead of days. Here, the authors discuss the effectiveness and complications of brachytherapy in STS, with a review of the pertinent literature.

Chapter 10 - Gallbladder carcinoma has an extremely bad prognosis. The radical surgery is acceptable for minority of patients; external radiotherapy or chemotherapy is ineffective. The aim of study was to evaluate the therapeutic effect of a combination of intraluminal brachytherapy (ILBT) and metallic stent implantation in the treatment of patients with nonresectable biliary tumours.

43 patients aged 41-80 years with nonresectable biliary malignancies - gallbladder carcinoma (n=14), Klatskin´s tumour (n=25) and carcinoma of papilla Vateri (n=4) were treated with a combination of ILBT (Ir 192, high dose radiation, total dose 30 Gy) and metallic stent implantation (ELLA CS®). ILBT and stent insertion were performed through percutaneous drainage in all patients.

The mean survival in patients with gallbladder carcinoma was 219 days (range 86-609, median 190 days) in patients with Klatskin´s tumour 483 days (range 85-1223, median 436 days) and in patients with carcinoma of papilla Vateri 850 days (range 48-1518, median 917 days). The rate of 2-year survival in these groups was 0%, 20% and 50% respectively. The survival time differed significantly. The mean time of stent patency was 203, 434 and 850 days respectively. No complications related directly to ILBT were observed.

ILBT combined with percutaneous stent implantation is a safe method and appears to prolong survival in inoperable patients with Klatskin´s tumour and carcinoma of papilla Vateri. No similar effect was observed in patients with gallbladder carcinoma.

In: Brachytherapy
Editor: Leoni M. Fischer

ISBN: 978-1-61728-750-3
© 2011 Nova Science Publishers, Inc.

Chapter 1

The Efficacy of Modern Prostate LDR Brachytherapy as Monotherapy and Options for Salvage

Jonathan D. Schoenfeld[1] and Irving D. Kaplan[2]
[1]Harvard Radiation Oncology Program, Massacheusetts, USA
[2]Beth Israel Deaconess Medical Center, Israel

The increasingly routine use of prostate surface antigen (PSA)-based screening has led to the diagnosis of more patients with organ-confined prostate cancer. These localized cancers are routinely treated with radical prostatectomy, external beam radiation therapy or prostate brachytherapy. Prostate brachytherapy is an appealing treatment for reasons including patient convenience, a favorable toxicity profile and cost-effectiveness. Consequently, the utilization of brachytherapy is increasing, both in the United States and around the world. Although there are no randomized trials comparing the various treatment modalities, and long-term efficacy data are somewhat limited, the available evidence suggests that prostate brachytherapy achieves favorable results in lower risk patients that rivals those achieved with radical prostatectomy and external beam radiation therapy in terms of local control, prevention of biochemical relapse, and prevention of prostate cancer specific and overall mortality. As improved risk stratification and imaging modalities increase the accuracy with which patients with organ-confined disease can be identified, these results can be expected to improve. In addition to better patient selection, ensuring the proper dose is delivered also impacts the efficacy of treatment. Improved techniques such as three-dimensional intra-operative planning can increase the likelihood that a sufficient and homogenous dose is delivered to the entire prostate including all suspicious or known lesions identified by clinical exam, imaging and prostate biopsy. In part due to these diagnostic and technical advancements, prostate brachytherapy may be an effective treatment for localized intermediate-risk disease, both as monotherapy and in combination with external beam radiation therapy.

Although of concern, local recurrences after properly performed and adequately dosed prostate brachytherapy are rare. Salvage options for these local recurrences exist and include prostatectomy, repeat focal brachytherapy, cryotherapy and high frequency ultrasound (HIFU). The infrequency of local recurrences limits the experience with and the evaluation of these salvage modalities, but more recent series have demonstrated reduced toxicity rates and a significant percentage of patients with durable responses.

In conclusion, adequately dosed prostate brachytherapy has demonstrated efficacy in treating organ-localized prostate cancer. Ultimately, due to the indolent nature of many prostate cancers, even longer term follow up will be needed to further assess the technological advances that can be expected to improve patient selection, dose delivery and salvage treatments.

Introduction

The number of men who undergo prostate-specific antigen (PSA)-based screening for prostate cancer has dramatically increased since the late 1980s, increasing over twelve-fold from 1988 to 1991 [Potosky, Miller et al. 1995]. Subsequently, the proportion of patients diagnosed with early stage disease has increased. Recent data suggest that currently more than 60% of patients with prostate cancer are diagnosed with non-palpable disease, and almost half have disease that can be classified as low-risk [Partin, Mangold et al. 2001; Cooperberg, Moul et al. 2005]. Many of these patients have disease confined to within the prostate and are, therefore, candidates for targeted local therapy. Conventional treatments for organ-confined prostate cancer are radical prostatectomy or radiation therapy, delivered either using external beam radiation or interstitial brachytherapy. Although there have been no modern randomized controlled trials comparing surgery to radiation therapy, large series have suggested similar local, distant and overall prostate cancer control rates with the two treatments [D'Amico, Whittington et al. 1998].

Brachytherapy has been used to treat prostate cancer dating back to the early 1900s, when radium treatments were delivered using a transurethral catheter by Pasteau and Degrais [Bagshaw, Kaplan et al. 1993]. Early transperineal implants also used radium and were described starting in 1915 by Benjamin Stockwell Barringer at Memorial Hospital [Barringer 1924; Barringer 1938] and by Young and colleagues at Johns Hopkins University in the early 1920s. In the 1950s, Flocks and colleagues at the University of Iowa performed over one hundred gold-198 interstitial implants during open surgery [Holm 1997]. The first iodine-125 implants were reported from Memorial Sloan-Kettering Hospital in 1972 [Whitmore, Hilaris et. al. 1972]. These iodine-125 implants were also performed at the time of open surgery and guided by direct visualization and palpation of the prostate gland without the use of a template. Consequently, an imprecise and non-homogenous dose was delivered to the prostate and the long-term disease control rates of patients treated in this manner were suboptimal.

In the 1980s, Danish physicians developed techniques to plan prostate brachytherapy in advance using ultrasound mapping and templates to guide therapy[Holm 1997]. These innovations made it possible to deliver a more homogenous dose to the entire prostate with increased accuracy using a transperineal approach. Modern prostate brachytherapy has integrated additional techniques including three-dimensional ultrasound guidance of seed deployment, intra-operative planning and dosimetry and, more recently, CT- or MRI-guided radiation planning. Increasing experience with these technologies allows for the targeted delivery of a high dose of radiation to the prostate gland and small surrounding margin with an increased sparing of adjacent normal tissue, most notably the bladder and bowel.

Table 1. Isotopes commonly used in LDR prostate brachytherapy

	Iodine-125	Palladium-103
Energy	27 keV x-ray	21 keV x-ray
Half-life	59.6 days	17 days
Approximate activity per seed	0.37 - 0.45 mCi	1.3 - 1.5 mCi

Currently, most prostate brachytherapy procedures in the United States are performed on an outpatient basis using permanent interstitial implants inserted through the perineum under general anesthesia. These permanent implants typically consist of small iodine-125 or palladium-103 radioactive seeds that deliver low-dose-rate treatment (LDR) of less than 40 cGy per hour to the prostate over weeks to months (Table 1). High dose rate (HDR) treatments of greater than 1200 cGy per hour have also been increasingly used and usually involve the placement of temporary prostate catheters from which radiation sources can be placed and removed. Consequently, HDR therapy usually requires a short hospitalization as patients receive several treatments over a few days.

Typically, prostate brachytherapy is either delivered as monotherapy or given as a radiation boost after external beam radiation therapy. When used as monotherapy, brachytherapy is most appropriate for patients who have a high probability of organ-localized disease because of the relatively steep dose gradient that exists in the peri-prostatic tissue. Thus, in the past, the limited numbers of patients diagnosed with early stage disease and the absence of accurate risk stratification limited the number of patients that could be identified as good candidates for brachytherapy as monotherapy. PSA-based screening has increased the detection of early stage prostate cancer[Cooperberg, Moul et al. 2005], and refinements in risk stratification based on clinical stage, Gleason score and PSA [Partin, Mangold et al. 2001] have increased the ability to predict organ-confined disease. Additionally, improvements in imaging techniques such as endorectal ultrasound and prostate MRI have further improved patient selection. Recent improvements to prostate MRI in particular have enhanced resolution and increased the sensitivity and specificity with which prostate cancer can be detected [Lawrentschuk and Fleshner 2009].

Prostate brachytherapy is convenient, minimally invasive, and cost effective when compared to the other standard treatments for prostate cancer[Buron, Le Vu et al. 2007]. In contrast to external beam radiation therapy, prostate brachytherapy does not deliver radiation directly through the skin surface, and therefore the doses of radiation delivered to the normal tissues surrounding the prostate can be minimal. Unlike radical prostatectomy, prostate brachytherapy is typically performed as an outpatient procedure and can often be performed on older men with multiple medical comorbities that would be poor candidates for prostatectomy.

Although a detailed discussion of morbidity following prostate brachytherapy is beyond the scope of this chapter, the toxicity profile of modern prostate brachytherapy is favorable. A recent study utilizing validated patient questionnaires obtained both before and after therapy[Sanda, Dunn et al. 2008] reported that only 1-5% of patients needed prolonged urinary catheterization after the procedure, with risk directly related to the size of the prostate gland and the degree to which urinary symptoms were present prior to treatment. The risk of erectile dysfunction varied with age, but potency was maintained in a majority of patients (approximately 79%) and erection-enhancing drugs were able to restore potency in the majority of patients (80%) in whom it was diminished after treatment. The rate of significant rectal toxicity was between 0-1%. Although there were inherent differences in patient selection, the toxicities associated with brachytherapy compared well with either radical prostatectomy or external beam radiation therapy.

The increase in eligible patients diagnosed with early-stage prostate cancer and the growing experience of physicians performing prostate brachytherapy has provided the impetus for a dramatic rise in the number of brachytherapy procedures performed in the United States and the rest of the world. In the United States, for example, data from an multi-institutional observational database of men with prostate cancer demonstrate a gradual increase in the percentage of prostate cancer patients treated with prostate brachytherapy from 3.4% to 5.3% from 1989 to 1998, and then a more rapid rise until brachytherapy accounted for the treatment of 13.1% of all patients diagnosed from 1999 to 2001 [Cooperberg, Grossfeld et al. 2003]. The overall use of brachytherapy for any malignancy increased in nineteen European countries by approximately 11% from 1997-2002, with 16% of those patients receiving prostate brachytherapy [Guedea, Ellison et al. 2007]. Japan introduced permanent iodine-125 implants in 2003, and already over 90 institutions have treated over 10,000 patients in this manner [Yoshioka 2009]. Surveys conducted in 1995 and 2000 in Australia and New Zealand demonstrate a significant increase in specialists who recommended prostate brachytherapy for organ-localized disease, although still significantly less than the number of physicians who recommended radical prostatectomy or external beam radiation therapy[Chong, Austen et al. 2006].

As interest in prostate brachytherapy increases, important considerations for both patients and physicians include the efficacy of this procedure and the options for local salvage when necessary.

Efficacy

Prostate cancer is often a slowly progressive disease, and thus it can take years and even decades for treatments to demonstrate a survival benefit [Bill-Axelson, Holmberg et al. 2008]. Consequently, prostate cancer studies often use the surrogate endpoint of biochemical failure (a significant rise in PSA following treatment) as a preliminary means to evaluate and compare the efficacy of potential therapies. Biochemical failure is associated with local failure [Stone, Stock et al. 2007], the development of distant metastases and prostate cancer death [Pound, Partin et al. 1999]. Unfortunately, various definitions of biochemical failure have been used as the sensitivity and experience with PSA testing has increased (Table 2), making it more challenging to compare published studies [Roach, Hanks et al. 2006]. Two common definitions of biochemical failure are generally used, the American Society for Therapeutic Radiation and Oncology (ASTRO) consensus 1997 definition and the ASTRO Phoenix (Nadir + 2 ng/ml) definition, although the ASTRO Phoenix definition is more sensitive and specific [Thames, Kuban et al. 2003]. The increased sensitivity and specificity of the Phoenix definition has also been confirmed specifically for brachytherapy patients [Kuban, Levy et al. 2006].

No modern prospective randomized trials have directly compared the efficacy of radical prostatectomy, external beam radiation therapy and brachytherapy [D'Amico, Whittington et al. 1998]. Attempts have been made to conduct such trials, for example by the Southwest Oncology Group in the 1980s and a more recently in low-risk prostate cancer patients in Canada, but all have had to close because of poor accrual [Klein, Ciezki et al. 2008]. Consequently, the efficacy of prostate brachytherapy has been estimated using single and multi-institutional series. In some cases, attempts have been made to directly compare efficacy results with prostate cancer patients that have undergone radical prostatectomy or external beam radiation as their primary treatment. However, these comparisons are limited by inherent bias in patient selection, although some studies have endeavored to account for this by comparing the results from equivalently risk-stratified patients.

Current guidelines for the risk stratification of prostate cancer patients categorize patients as low, intermediate and high risk [National Comprehensive Cancer Network 2009]. These risk groups are based on the established risk factors: PSA-level, clinical stage and Gleason score - factors that have been demonstrated to predict for the pathologic extent of disease and for prognosis following treatment [Partin, Mangold et al. 2001]. However, these risk groups are limited in that they do not take other prognostic factors into account: age, medical comorbidities, PSA-velocity, percent positive cores identified at biopsy, presence of perineural invasion, imaging results, among others[D'Amico, Renshaw et al. 2004; D'Amico, Renshaw et al. 2005; Beard, Schultz et al. 2006]. Thus, there is significant heterogeneity within each risk group. Furthermore, the risk groups have changed over time and are not uniform among different centers, limiting the ability to compare between studies (Table 3). Nevertheless, stratifying patients into risk groups based on prognostic factors remains useful when examining efficacy data from published studies.

Improved risk stratification, innovations in brachytherapy technique, increased experience and combined modality therapy are likely to have improved the efficacy of prostate brachytherapy. More sophisticated risk stratification has improved patient selection and allowed for the treatment of particular subgroups of patients that may not have otherwise been eligible. Improved technology has allowed for the delivery of a higher, more homogenous and more accurately targeted radiation dose to be delivered to the prostate. Prostate brachytherapy has also been combined with androgen deprivation therapy and external beam radiation therapy, although combinations with these other treatments make comparisons among previous published series more difficult to interpret (Table 2). Androgen deprivation therapy, in particular, is often given prior to prostate brachytherapy in order to downsize the prostate, although in some series it is has also been used after brachytherapy in intermediate- or high-risk patients.

Table 2. Variable definitions of biochemical failure, use of androgen deprivation therapy and use of external beam radiation therapy in series evaluating prostate brachytherapy

Study	Biochemical Failure	Androgen Deprivation	EBRT
Beyer 2000	ASTRO	None	None
Block 2006	ASTRO	58.50%	None
D'Amico 1998	ASTRO	In specified subgroup	In specified subgroup
Grimm 2001	Two consecutive PSA rises	None	None
Guedea 2006	ASTRO	38.60%	None
Henry 2010	ASTRO and Phoenix	44% (neoadjuvant only)	None
Hinnen 2009	Phoenix	9.20%	None
Khaksar 2006	ASTRO	66%	22%
Klein 2008	One value > 0.3 ng/ml for RP; Phoenix for EBRT or BT	None	None
Kupelian 2004	Two values >0.2 ng/ml for RP; ASTRO for EBRT or BT	21% (neoadjuvant only)	In specified subgroup
Mitchell 2008	ASTRO and Phoenix	26.30%	3.50%
Morris 2009	Phoenix	65%	None
Potters 2005	ASTRO, Phoenix, ASTRO-Kattan, ASTRO-Last call	19.20%	12.40%
Ragde 2000	ASTRO	None	36%
Stone 2007	ASTRO-Kattan and Phoenix	39.20%	22.50%
Stone 2005	ASTRO	27.60%	None
Taira 2009	One value > 0.4 ng/ml after nadir	None	None
Zelefsky, Yamada 2007	ASTRO and Phoenix	35% (noeadjuvant only)	None
Zelefsky, Kuban 2007	ASTRO and Phoenix	None	None

ASTRO: three consecutive rises, backdated.
ASTRO-Kattan: three rises, not necessarily consecutive.
ASTRO-Last call: three increases, not backdated.
Phoenix: PSA nadir + 2 ng/ml.
RP: radical prostatectomy
EBRT: external beam radiation therapy
BT: prostate brachytherapy

Table 3. Variable risk group definitions used in series evaluating prostate brachytherapy

Study	Low-risk	Intermediate-risk	High-risk
Block 2006	PSA<10, Gleason<=6, T1b-2a	None	None
D'Amico 1998	PSA<=10, Gleason<=6, T1c-T2a	PSA 10-20, Gleason 7 or T2b	PSA>20, Gleason>7 or T2c
Guedea 2006	PSA<=10, Gleason<=6, T1-T2b	Either PSA>10, Gleason>6 or stage>=T2c	Two or more intermediate factors
Henry 2010	PSA<10, Gleason <=6, T1-T2	Either PSA>10, Gleason>6 or T3	Two or more intermediate factors or PSA>20,
Hinnen 2009	PSA<10, Gleason<=6, T1b-2a	Either PSA 10-20, Gleason 7 or T2b-T2c	Gleason>7 or T3
Khaksar 2006	PSA<10, Gleason<=6, T1-T2b	Either PSA>10, Gleason>6 or stage>=T2c	Two or more intermediate factors
Klein 2008	None	Undefined	None
Morris 2009	PSA<10, Gleason<=6, T1-T2b	Low-tier intermediate: Stage<T3 and either PSA<=10 and Gleason 7 or PSA 10-15 and Gleason<=6	None
Potters 2005	PSA<10, Gleason<=6, <50% of cores positive	Either PSA>10, Gleason>=7 or >50% cores positive	Two or more intermediate factors or PSA>20,
Stone 2007	PSA<10, Gleason<=6, T1b-2a	Either PSA 10-20, Gleason 7 or T2b-T2c	Gleason>7 or T3
Stone 2005	PSA<=10, Gleason<=6, T1-2a	None	All others
Taira 2009	PSA<10, Gleason<=6, T1-T2b	Either PSA 10-20, Gleason 7 or T2c	None
Zelefsky, Yamada 2007	PSA<10, Gleason<=6, T1b-2a	Either PSA 10-20, Gleason 7 or T2b-T2c	PSA>20, Gleason>=8 or T3
Zelefsky, Kuban 2007	PSA<10, Gleason<=6, T1b-2a	Either PSA 10-20, Gleason 7 or T2b-T2c	PSA>20 or Gleason>=8

PSA (ng/ml)

T1b: Incidental finding in >5% of tissue.

T1c: PSA detected, non-palpable

T2a: Tumor involving less than 1/2 of one lobe

T2b: Tumor involving one lobe

T2c: Tumor involving both lobes

T3: Tumor extends beyond the prostatic capsule

Comparisons with Radical Prostatectomy and External Beam Radiation Therapy

Although there are no randomized controlled trials comparing prostate brachytherapy with other treatment modalities, large retrospective studies in the modern era have suggested that well selected patients with low- to intermediate-risk disease fare as well after brachytherapy as they do after radical prostatectomy or external beam therapy (Table 4). Some earlier studies did suggest worse outcomes after brachytherapy, but often these studies did not correct for significant selection biases, disregarding risk factors such as tumor stage [Polascik, Pound et al. 1998]. Additionally, uniform definitions of biochemical failure were often used after radical prostatectomy and prostate brachytherapy, even though it is now known that patients can have a temporary PSA "bounce" following prostate irradiation that is not predictive of outcome [Horwitz, Levy et al. 2006]. Even considering these deficiencies, some early comparisons where an attempt was made to evaluate and compare efficacy results of risk-stratified patients did not find a significant difference in recurrence free survival between radical prostatectomy and prostate brachytherapy [Ramos, Carvalhal et al. 1999].

One of the largest studies to risk-stratify prostate cancer patients and compare outcomes after therapy was a retrospective cohort analysis of 1872 men treated between 1989 and 1997 with radical prostatectomy or prostate brachytherapy performed at the Hospital of the University of Pennsylvania or external beam radiation therapy performed at the Joint Center for Radiation Therapy in Boston [D'Amico, Whittington et al. 1998]. Prostate brachytherapy used palladium-103 seeds with a minimum peripheral dose to the prostate of 115 Gy. The median follow up was 38-41 months for patients treated with the various modalities (range 8-100). For low-risk patients, the relative risk of biochemical failure at five years was not significantly different among patients treated with radical prostatectomy, external beam radiation or brachytherapy. Furthermore, all treatment modalities resulted in a greater than 80% freedom from biochemical failure at five years for patients with low-risk disease. Both intermediate- and high-risk patients treated with brachytherapy alone had a significantly increased risk of biochemical failure compared with those patients treated with radical prostatectomy (relative risks of 3.1 and 3.0, respectively), although intermediate-risk patients treated with brachytherapy combined with androgen deprivation therapy were not at an increased risk. The absolute rates of biochemical failure at five years for intermediate-risk patients treated with brachytherapy alone were 60-70%, compared to less than 50% with the other treatment modalities. Finally, all patients with high-risk disease treated with prostate brachytherapy demonstrated biochemical failure with five years of follow up, although results with radical prostatectomy and external beam therapy were also poor.

Table 4. Select series directly comparing prostate brachytherapy to other treatment modalities

D'Amico 1998 (n = 1872)					
Relative risk of biochemical failure following:	RP (n = 888)	EBRT (n = 766)	BT monotherapy (n = 66)	BT and ADT (n = 152)	
Median follow-up, months	38	38	41	41	
Low-risk patients (95% Confidence Interval)	1	1.1 (0.5-2.7)	1.1 (0.3-3.6)	0.5 (0.1-1.9)	
Intermediate-risk patients	1	0.8 (0.5-1.2)	3.1 (1.5-6.1)	1.6 (0.8-3.3)	
High-risk patients	1	0.9 (0.7-1.1)	3 (1.8-5)	2.2 (1.2-4)	
Kupelian 2004 (n = 2991)	RP (n = 1034)	EBRT <72 Gy (n = 484)	EBRT >72 Gy (n = 301)	BT (n = 950)	EBRT + BT (n = 222)
Median follow-up, months	66	75	49	47	46
Biochemical relapse-fee survival (at 5-years)	81%	51%	81%	83%	77%
Klein 2008 (n = 861, all intermediate-risk)	RP (n = 336)	EBRT (n = 321)	BT (n = 204)		
Median follow up, months	59%	58%	39%		
Biochemical relapse-free survival (at 5 years), p = .052	76%	80%	82%		
Clinical failure free survival (at 5 years), p = .188	98%	95%	97%		
Overall survival, (at 5 years) p = .046	98%	93%	94%		
Beyer 2000 (n = 2222), Failure free survival at 5 years	EBRT (n = 1527)	BT (n = 695)			
Median follow up, months	41.3	51.3			
Overall, p = 0.91	69%	71%			
Patients with Gleason scores 8-10, p = .04	52%	28%			
Patients with initial PSA 10-20 ng/ml	70%	53%			

RP: radical prostatectomy
EBRT: external beam radiation therapy
BT: brachytherapy
ADT: androgen deprivation therapy

Table 5. Institutional series evaluating the efficacy of prostate brachytherapy

	n (low-, intermediate-, high-risk)	Median follow-up	Results at:	Low-risk	Intermediate-risk	High-risk	All patients
Biochemical relapse-free survival							
Block 2006	118 (118, 0, 0)	48.9 months	5 years	94.7%			94.7%
Grimm 2001	125	82 months	10 years	87%			85.1%
Guedea 2006	1050 (668, 297, 66)	Unknown	3 years	93%	88%	80%	91%
Hinnen 2009	921 (232, 369, 320)	69 months	10 years	88%	61%	30%	57%
Khaksar 2006	300 (146, 111, 43)	45 months	5 years	96%	89%	93%	93%
Mitchell 2008	1535	21 months	3 years				94.4% (ASTRO) 94.5% (Phoenix)
Morris 2009	1006	54 months	5 years				95.6%
Potters 2005	1449 (481, 554, 418)	82 months	12 years	91% (ASTRO) 89% (ASTRO-Kattan) 85% (ASTRO-Last call) 88% (Phoenix)	80% (ASTRO) 78% (ASTRO-Kattan) 74% (ASTRO-Last call) 76% (Phoenix)	66% (ASTRO) 63% (ASTRO-Kattan) 59% (ASTRO-Last call) 62% (Phoenix)	81% (ASTRO) 78% (ASTRO-Kattan) 74% (ASTRO-Last call) 77% (Phoenix)
Ragde 2000	147	122 months	10 years				66%
Stone 2005	279	72 months	10 years	91%			78%
Stone 2007	3928 (2188, 1188, 552)	42.5 months	10 years	84.1% (ASTRO-Kattan) 78.1% (Phoenix)	76.8% (ASTRO-Kattan) 63.6% (Phoenix)	64.4% (ASTRO-Kattan) 58.2% (Phoenix)	79.2% (ASTRO-Kattan) 70% (Phoenix)
Taira 2009	463 (319, 144, 0)	69.6 months	12 years	97.4%	96.4%		97.1%
Zelefsky, Kuban 2007	2693 (1444, 960, 192)	63 months	8 years	82% (ASTRO) 74% (Phoenix)	70% (ASTRO) 61% (Phoenix)	48% (ASTRO) 39% (Phoenix)	
Zelefsky, Yamada 2007	367 (319, 47, 1)	63 months	5 years	96% (ASTRO) 96% (Phoenix)	90% (ASTRO) 88% (Phoenix)		
Metastasis-free survival							
Grimm 2001	125	82 months	10 years				96.8%
Morris 2009	1006	54 months	5 years				99%
Zelefsky, Kuban 2007	2693 (1444, 960, 192)	63 months	8 years	98%	92%	85%	
Cancer-specific survival							
Hinnen 2009	921 (232, 369, 320)	69 months	10 years	96%	87%	69%	82%

Study	N						
Potters 2005	1449 (481, 554, 418)	82 months	12 years				93%
Ragde 2000	147	122 months	10 years				70%
Taira 2009	463 (319, 144, 0)	69.6 months	12 years	99.6%	100%		99.7%
Overall survival							
Grimm 2001	125	82 months	10 years				
Hinnen 2009	921 (232, 369, 320)	69 months	10 years	68%	64%	49%	59%
Morris 2009	1006	66 months	5 years				95.2%
Potters 2005	1449 (481, 554, 418)	82 months	12 years				81%
Taira 2009	463 (319, 144, 0)	69.6 months	12 years	76.2%	74%		75.4%
Zelefsky, Kuban 2007	2693 (1444, 960, 192)	63 months	8 years	81%	71%	63%	63%

ASTRO: three consecutive rises, backdated.

ASTRO-Kattan: three rises, not necessarily consecutive.

ASTRO-Last call: three increases, not backdated.

Phoenix: PSA nadir + 2 ng/ml.

This retrospective cohort analysis is one of the few series that has directly compared the efficacy of various prostate cancer treatments in risk-stratified patients. Unfortunately, however, only 66 patients in this cohort were treated with prostate brachytherapy alone, limiting the conclusions that can be drawn from these results. Additionally, the only comparisons that were made were based on biochemical failure with no reporting of survival data.

Kupelian et. al. [Kupelian, Potters et al. 2004] examined the rates of biochemical relapse in 2991 clinically localized prostate cancer patients treated between 1990 and 1998 at the Cleveland Clinic Foundation or Memorial Sloan Kettering at Mercy Medical Center with radical prostatectomy, external beam radiation and radiation. With a median follow up of 56 months (range 12-145 months), biochemical relapse-free survival at five years was 81% in patients treated with radical prostatectomy, 51% in patients treated with external beam radiation therapy to doses less than 72 Gy, 81% for patients treated with external beam radiation therapy to doses greater than 72 Gy, 83% for patients treated with brachytherapy alone, and 77% for patients treated with external beam radiation therapy combined with a brachytherapy boost. As expected, there were significant differences among the patients who received the various treatments in terms of their pretreatment PSA levels, Gleason score and clinical stage. However, in a proportional hazards multivariable model excluding the low dose external beam radiotherapy group and evaluating the use of androgen deprivation, treatment modality, T-stage, PSA, Gleason score and year of therapy, treatment modality was not a significant predictor of biochemical relapse free survival.

An analysis limited to intermediate-risk patients in the Localized Prostate Cancer Database was performed on 861 patients treated from 1996 to 2004 at the Cleveland Clinic [Klein, Ciezki et al. 2008]. Prostate brachytherapy was performed using iodine-125 seeds prescribed to a dose of 144 Gy. With a median follow up of 39, 59 and 58 months for patients treated with brachytherapy, radical prostatectomy and external beam radiation therapy, respectively, there were no differences in the rates of biochemical failure. Although there was a small difference in clinical recurrence-free survival and overall survival favoring the radical prostatectomy patients, there were very few clinical failures (less than 15 patients overall), most of which represented metastatic disease. Less than 2% of all patients died of prostate cancer.

A retrospective comparison limited to comparing the efficacy of external beam radiation and brachytherapy in 2222 patients treated from 1988 to 1995 was conducted at a multiphysician radiation oncologist practice in the metropolitan Phoenix area with data maintained in the Arizona Oncology Services database[Beyer and Brachman 2000; Brachman, Thomas et al. 2000]. The median age of the patients was 74 years and the median follow-up was 41.3 and 51.3 months for the patients treated with external beam radiation and brachytherapy, respectively. EBRT was delivered to a mean total dose of 66.6 Gy and brachytherapy was performed with iodine-125 seeds prescribed to 160 Gy in 663 patients and palladium-103 seeds prescribed to 120 Gy in 32 patients. This study demonstrated that both modalities were equally effective at maintaining failure-free survival at five years (69% for EBRT, 71% for BT). However, subgroup analyses revealed that patients with Gleason 8-10 tumors and pretreatment PSA levels between 10-20 ng/ml fared significantly better after EBRT compared with brachytherapy.

Institutional Series

Many multi- or single institution series of patients treated with brachytherapy as monotherapy have achieved durable and long-term biochemical recurrence free survival after treatment (Table 5). Low-risk patients, in particular, have demonstrated durable biochemical control rates generally greater than 75% in the largest modern trials with follow-up longer than ten years. Although sometimes used as monotherapy, brachytherapy has also been used in combination with hormones or external beam radiation therapy to treat intermediate or high-risk patients due to the higher rates of failure observed with brachytherapy alone. High-risk patients have a significant risk of disease that has escaped the prostate gland. Consequently, in recent years less than 3% of all high-risk patients have received brachytherapy as monotherapy, despite the overall nation-wide trend towards performing more brachytherapy procedures [Cooperberg, Grossfeld et al. 2003].

One of the largest published multi-institutional series of prostate cancer patients treated with brachytherapy as monotherapy includes 2,693 patients treated at 11 American institutions from 1988 to 1998 [Zelefsky, Kuban et al. 2007]. All patients had clinically localized (T1-T2) prostate cancer and none received androgen deprivation therapy before PSA-failure. With a median follow up of 63 months (range 4-180 months), low-risk patients had an eight-year biochemical-relapse free survival of 74%-82% depending on the definition of biochemical failure used. Intermediate-risk and high-risk patients had eight-year biochemical-relapse free survivals of 61-70% and 39-48%, respectively. The eight-year distant metastases-free, clinical disease-free, and overall survival rates were all high and generally comparable to results from series of patients treated with radical prostatectomy and external beam radiation therapy. Tumor stage, Gleason score, pretreatment PSA, and year of treatment all significantly impacted the probability of biochemical failure-free survival. Finally, results were better among patients whose dosimetry information was available and who had an increased dose delivered to 90% of the prostate.

A partially overlapping series of 3928 patients treated with brachytherapy at six centers in the United States also obtained favorable results [Stone, Potters et al. 2007]. With a median follow up of 42.5 months (range 1.8-161 months), the ten-year biochemical failure free survival was 78-84% for low-risk patients, 64-77% for intermediate-risk patients and 58-64% for high risk patients.

A European multi-institutional series was reported with the results from 1050 localized prostate cancer patients treated with prostate brachytherapy at 5 European centers in France, Finland, Italy, Spain and the United Kingdom from 1998-2003 [Guedea, Aguilo et al. 2006]. With 364 patients having follow-up over 3 years, the 3-year rates of biochemical relapse-free survival was 93% for low-risk patients, 88% for intermediate-risk patients and 80% for high-risk patients.

A prospectively compiled database of 1535 patients treated with iodine-125 implants at three institutions in the United Kingdom from 2003-2006 demonstrated a two-year biochemical failure-free survival of greater than 94% with a median follow-up of 21 months (range 1 – 56 months) [Mitchell, Mandall et al. 2008]. One hundred fifty-nine men with intermediate- or high-risk disease and 228 men with enlarged prostates also received androgen deprivation therapy. In an update on a subset of these patients treated at one of the participating institutions, overall biochemical failure-free survival with a median follow-up of

4.9 years (range 2.03 – 11.7 years) was over 72% at 10 years, overall-survival was 85%, and disease-specific survival was 95% [Henry, Al-Qaisieh et al. 2010].

Single institution series have also demonstrated favorable results for low-risk prostate cancer patients treated with brachytherapy as monotherapy. Treating 125 consecutive and predominantly low-risk patients from 1988 to 1990 with iodine-125 implants, the Seattle Prostate Institute reported a ten-year biochemical control rate of 85% with a median follow-up of 82 months [Grimm, Blasko et al. 2001]. For 463 patients treated for clinically localized prostate cancer from 1995-2005 with prostate brachytherapy at the Schiffler Cancer Center in Wheeling, West Virginia with a median follow-up of 5.8 years, twelve-year biochemical progression-free survival was 97.1% [Taira, Merrick et al. 2009]. Cause-specific and overall survival rates were 99.7% and 75.4%, respectively.

Other series from single institutions have combined brachytherapy with other treatments, making the results more difficult to interpret (Table 2). The results for 1449 consecutive prostate cancer patients treated with brachytherapy from 1992 to 2000 were reported in 2005 [Potters, Morgenstern et al. 2005], 400 who also received androgen deprivation therapy and 301 who were also treated with external beam radiation therapy. With a median follow-up of 82 months, the twelve-year biochemical relapse free survival rate was 74-81% with an overall survival of 81% and a disease-specific survival of 93%. The use of hormones or external beam radiation therapy in addition to brachytherapy may have influenced the results of this study; however, neither treatment significantly impacted biochemical control on multivariate analysis. From 1998-2002, 367 patients with low-risk or intermediate-risk prostate cancer were treated with intraoperatively planned iodine-125 implants at Memorial Sloan-Kettering Cancer Center [Zelefsky, Yamada et al. 2007]. Biochemical relapse-free survival at five years was 96% for the low-risk patients and 88-90% for the intermediate-risk patients. Although no patient received androgen deprivation therapy after brachytherapy and before biochemical relapse, patients with enlarged prostate glands greater than 50 ml in size generally received 3 months of androgen deprivation, although it had no significant impact on biochemical relapse-free survival. Stone et. al. [Stone, Stock et al. 2005] reported on 279 men treated with iodine-125 implants from 1990-1998, 64 of whom also received hormonal therapy before and after brachytherapy. With a median follow-up of six years (range 4-12 years), the ten-year biochemical failure-free survival was 78%. Additionally, repeat prostate biopsies were negative in 90% of the 185 patients in which they were performed.

Single institution series from international centers have also frequently combined androgen deprivation therapy with prostate brachytherapy. A Canadian series reported results from 1006 consecutive patients with low-risk or favorable intermediate-risk features treated with prostate brachytherapy from 1998-2003 [Morris, Keyes et al. 2009]. Most had also received androgen deprivation therapy. With a median follow-up of greater than 54 months, biochemical failure free-survival at five years was 95.6%, with the rate of distant metastases and disease specific survival both less than 1%. The rate of overall survival was 95%. A series of 118 low-risk patients treated in Germany from 1999-2002 had a five-year biochemical control rate of 94.7% with a median follow up of 48.9 months [Block, Czempiel et al. 2006]. Sixty-nine patients were treated with neoadjuvant androgen deprivation therapy. The University Medical Centre in Utrecht, The Netherlands treated 921 patients from 1989 to 2004 with iodine-125 implants, 85 of whom received six months of androgen deprivation prior to implant [Battermann, Boon et al. 2004; Hinnen, Battermann et al. 2009]. With a median follow-up of 69 months, there was an 88% biochemical recurrence-free survival at ten years and a disease specific survival of 82%.

Some older institutional series that formed the basis of early comparisons with other treatment modalities included combinations of brachytherapy with androgen deprivation therapy and external beam radiation therapy in select patients. One of these series consisted of 229 patients treated with iodine-125 implants at the Northwest Hospital in Seattle Washington from 1987-1989 [Ragde, Korb et al. 2000]. Eighty-two of these patients were deemed to be at increased risk of extracapsular disease and were treated with external beam radiation therapy in addition to brachytherapy. With a median follow-up of 122 months (range 18 – 144 months), ten-year disease-free survival was 70%, and was 66% in the patients that received brachytherapy alone. Disease-free survival was lower in this study compared with other brachytherapy series, potentially because these patients were treated immediately after the introduction of modern brachytherapy, as implantation techniques and dosimetry were evolving. These patients were also treated before PSA level was commonly used; thus, 80% were diagnosed with palpable disease, a far greater percentage than in most modern cohorts.

Evolving Trends

Improvements in technology and the growing experience with prostate brachytherapy have increased the ability to ensure that a more homogeneous dose is consistently delivered. Evidence suggests that this consistency has increased the efficacy of prostate brachytherapy [Grimm, Blasko et al. 2001; Battermann, Boon et al. 2004]. Additionally, more precise dosimetry has increased the potential for dose escalation or for specific targeting of higher doses to areas of known disease. Furthermore, as techniques have improved, there has been more willingness to investigate the use of brachytherapy in particular subgroups of patients that were not initially thought to be ideal candidates for the procedure, i.e. younger patients or select patients with intermediate risk disease. Many series described below have now demonstrated promising early efficacy rates for these patients.

Dosimetry

The dose prescribed in prostate brachytherapy varies with the particular isotope used and has varied over time. Improved dose homogeneity and target delineation have resulted from the increasing use of more sophisticated image guided techniques. The Seattle Prostate Institute popularized a preplanning approach whereby transrectal ultrasound images obtained prior to the brachytherapy procedure allowed a treatment planning system to generate the seed-loading pattern based on calculated dose distributions. Patients who underwent preplanning had better outcomes than patients with no planning [Battermann, Boon et al. 2004] and, consequently, treatment era became a predictive factor for outcome [Hinnen, Battermann et al. 2009]. More recently, the use of intra-operative planning using transrectal ultrasound (Figure 1) allows the physician and dosimetrist to ensure that the planning position is identical to the treatment position [Zelefsky, Yamada et al. 2000]. By continuing to monitor the position of the placed seeds in real time, adjustments can be made for variation in prostate geometry caused by subtle changes in patient anatomy or by the placement of prior seeds.

Furthermore, intra-operative planning allows for immediate confirmation of seed placement and, if needed, for adjustments based on variability in the position of previously placed seeds. Combining axial and sagittal imaging with ultrasound allows for the accurate localization of each seed in three-dimensional space and therefore can ensure that the dose delivered to bladder and urethra is minimized as much possible while not compromising dose to the prostate (Figure 2). Indeed, intraoperative imaging and planning provides the flexibility to ensure that areas with suspicious lesions or biopsy proven-disease will receive an adequate or even an increased dose (Figure 3).

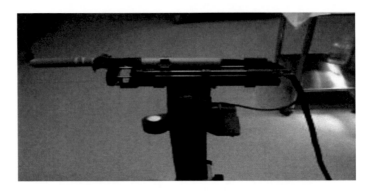

Figure 1. Typical transrectal ultrasound set-up.

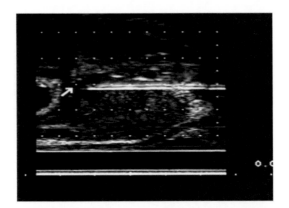

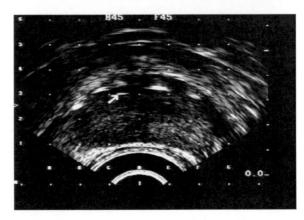

Figure 2. Intra-operative localization of seed placement in three-dimensional space.

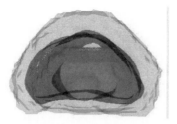 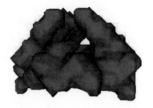

Figure 3. Sample dose cloud generated by intra-operative planning.

With these modern techniques, higher doses, specifically those greater than 140 Gy when iodine-125 is used, have resulted in increased biochemical control rates [Stock, Stone et al. 1998]. Indeed, the retrospective series reported by Stone et. al. [2005] identified a three-fold risk of biochemical failure rate for brachytherapy patients who received doses to 90% of the prostate (D90) of less than 140 Gy ($p<0.01$) and a 5.6-fold increased risk of failure for patients with a D90 less than 120 Gy ($p<0.01$). In low-risk patients, the eight-year biochemical relapse-free survival was 94% in patients who received an optimal dose (D90 for iodine-125 seeds of greater than 140 Gy or greater than 115 Gy for palladium-103 seeds) compared with a 75% biochemical relapse-free survival for those whose dosimetry was suboptimal ($p = 0.02$) [Kollmeier, Stock et al. 2003]. An improved biochemical recurrence-free survival of 88% compared with 78% at ten years was also observed with a D90 of greater than 140 Gy in a contemporary series from the United Kingdom[Henry, Al-Qaisieh et al. 2010]. Finally, there is some evidence that even higher doses may lead to improved efficacy in certain patients. Patients treated to doses greater than 180 Gy at Mt. Sinai School of Medicine demonstrated a greater than 95% biochemical relapse-free survival at 5-years, with intermediate and high-risk patients notably demonstrating greater than 90% biochemical relapse-free survival [Kao, Stone et al. 2008].

The homogeneity of the dose delivered to the prostate also affects outcomes. Patients who receive 100% of the prescribed dose to less than 90% of the prostate have been shown to have a decreased biochemical relapse-free survival[Wallner, Merrick et al. 2005]. Similarly, the importance of adequate D90 was noted in multivariate analysis performed on patients treated in the series reported by Potters et. al. [2005].

Assessing the adequacy and homogeneity of prior brachytherapy treatments is even more difficult when the different methods that have been used to evaluate brachytherapy dosimetry are considered. Many prior studies focused on the minimal peripheral dose delivered to the prostate based on plain films [Ragde, Korb et al. 2000], even though plain films provide only a rough estimation of actual prostate volume and location. Current guidelines issued by the American Brachytherapy Society focus on the D90 as determined by CT scan performed after the procedure [Nag, Bice et al. 2000], even though ultrasound imaging is generally used intraoperatively and the prostate is known to change shape following brachytherapy due to the edema that results from the procedure (Figure 4) (Zelefsky, Yamada et al. 2007).

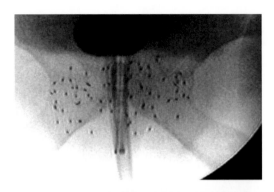

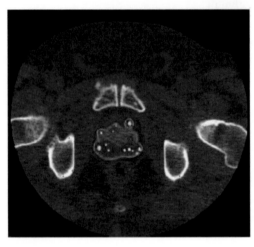

Figure 4. Currently, seed placement is confirmed with plain films, while dosimetry is performed with the aid of postoperative CT scans.

Although achieving adequate and homogenous dose clearly impacts on efficacy, more recent studies that have been able to control for dose delivered have not demonstrated a difference in the efficacy of brachytherapy when either of the two most commonly used isotopes are used: iodine-125 and palladium-103. For example, the multi-institutional study reported by Zelefsky and colleagues demonstrated a 93% eight-year biochemical relapse-free survival for patients treated with iodine-125 where the dose delivered to 90% of the prostate was greater than 130 Gy, compared with 76% for patients where the dose delivered to 90% of the prostate was less than 130 Gy [Zelefsky, Kuban et al. 2007]. Similarly, for patients treated with palladium-103, the five-year biochemical relapse-free survival was 92% for patients that received greater or equal than 115 Gy to 90% of the prostate compared with 83% for patients that received less than 115 Gy. Although isotope used significantly affected outcome on initial multivariable analysis, it no longer had a significant effect when the dose effect was taken into account. Likewise, a study that randomized 126 patients to either iodine-125 or palladium-103 implants did not observe differences in outcomes [Wallner, Merrick et al. 2003].

Patient selection

Because of the focality of prostate brachytherapy treatment, the ideal brachytherapy candidate has organ-confined disease. Unfortunately, determining which patients have localized disease is difficult prior to therapy. Historically, the digital rectal exam was used in isolation to identify the presence of extraprostatic disease, although digital exam alone likely misclassified approximately half of all patients with extracapsular extention as having organ-confined disease [Kattan, Stapleton et al. 1997]. More recently, factors such as Gleason score and PSA level have been combined with the clinical exam to risk-stratify patients and better estimate the risks of disease spread [Kattan, Stapleton et al. 1997; Partin, Mangold et al. 2001]. However, limiting brachytherapy to only the low-risk patients may exclude more than 60% of intermediate-risk patients with organ confined disease [Lieberfarb, Schultz et al. 2002], while treating more than 2% of low-risk patients with disease that has already spread beyond the prostate. Improvements in imaging technology, most notably the development of a pelvic MRI performed with the use of an endorectal coil placed adjacent to the prostate has sought to improve risk-stratification by identifying additional patients with organ-confined disease who may therefore be amenable to prostate brachytherapy (Figure 5). Evidence suggests that modern pelvic MRI can identify extraprostatic cancer approximately 67-100% of the time [Turkbey, Pinto et al. 2009] and may be the most sensitive predictor of pathologic extension of disease outside the prostate [D'Amico, Whittington et al. 1996].

With the use of improved risk-stratification and dosimetry, subgroup analyses have suggested that well-selected intermediate-risk or even high-risk patients may have favorable long-term prostate cancer control after brachytherapy as monotherapy. In a classification and regression tree analysis conducted on patients treated with palladium-103 with doses delivered to 90% of the prostate greater than 115 Gy, patients with Gleason scores of 7-10 included in the large multi-institutional series reported by Zelefsky et. al. achieved an eight-year PSA-progression free survival of 82% [Zelefsky, Kuban et al. 2007]. Similarly, a multi-center review of 5889 patients with Gleason score 7-10 disease demonstrated an increased biochemical relapse-free survival of over 88% and a decreased rate of metastatic events at five years when increased radiation doses were given either with brachytherapy alone or a combination of brachytherapy and external beam radiation therapy[Stone, Stock et al. 2009]. The benefit of increased dose on biochemical control in both intermediate and high-risk patients was also noted in an earlier study [Stone, Potters et al. 2007]. Another retrospective study that compared brachytherapy monotherapy to brachytherapy plus external beam radiation did not find any evidence of added benefit to adding external beam radiation in the treatment of intermediate-risk patients, suggesting that brachytherapy monotherapy could provide adequate treatment [Merrick, Butler et al. 2005]. The high eight-year biochemical relapse-free survival rate of over 95% demonstrated in patients treated with brachytherapy monotherapy in this study also provided evidence of the increased efficacy of modern brachytherapy. Clearly, additional studies are warranted to further clarify which intermediate or even high-risk patients may potentially be appropriate candidates for brachytherapy as monotherapy, and the Radiation Therapy Oncology Group (RTOG) is currently conducting a trial examining the role of monotherapy versus combined therapy for intermediate-risk patients (RTOG 0232).

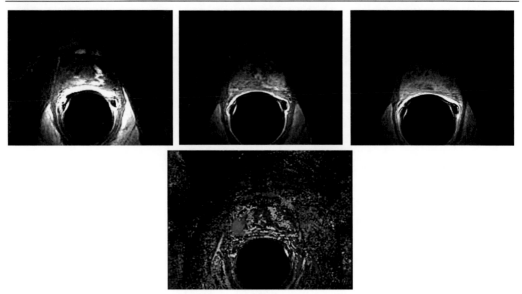

Figure 5. 3-Tesla endorectal MRI with Dynamic Contrast Enhancement. Red pixels represent areas of intermediate contrast kinetics. Blue pixels represent areas of slow contrast kinetics and correlate with normal prostate.

In addition to select intermediate and high-risk patients, prostate brachytherapy has demonstrated promising efficacy in other subgroups of patients that were previously infrequently treated. Younger patients have traditionally received prostate brachytherapy less frequently because of concerns regarding the long-term efficacy and toxicity of brachytherapy in this population. Merrick et. al., however, reported a series of 108 patients less than 54 years of age that were treated with brachytherapy, with 61 low-risk patients as treated with brachytherapy as monotherapy [Merrick, Wallner et al. 2006]. Overall eight-year biochemical relapse free survival with a median follow up of 4.8 years was 96%, and was also 96% for the 61 low-risk patients treated with brachytherapy as monotherapy. Similarly, an additional 119 patients less than 62 years-old treated with prostate brachytherapy (67 as monotherapy) had a seven-year biochemical failure free survival of 98.3% [Merrick, Butler et al. 2004]. Patients older than 75 years have also been treated successfully with prostate brachytherapy with greater than 97% biochemical relapse-free survival at nine years with a median follow-up of 5.8 years, although 55% of patients in this series received supplemental radiotherapy and 48% received androgen deprivation therapy of variable duration [Merrick, Wallner et al. 2008].

Salvage

Estimates for the percentage of patients that have local failures after prostate brachytherapy vary, but are around 10% in modern series [Stone, Stock et al. 2007; Stone, Stock et al. 2009]. Although the rate of local failure is low, some patients with a rising PSA after brachytherapy will have recurrence of disease isolated to within the prostate that can be identified on prostate imaging or on biopsy. Those patients where recurrence is likely limited to the prostate and with no evidence of metastatic disease are candidates for salvage therapy, with a goal of cure [Beyer 2003]. Options for local salvage treatments for these patients include radical prostatectomy, a second salvage brachytherapy procedure, focal cryotherapy, or high-frequency ultrasound. Although there has been reluctance to use these procedures because of historically increased toxicity rates [Sylvester, Grimm et al. 2001], androgen deprivation alone or no treatment does not provide an opportunity for cure. With increasing utilization of salvage procedures, more data have been accumulated regarding outcomes and modern toxicity rates. Outcome data for these procedures after brachytherapy are limited, however, because they have been most frequently used for salvage therapy following external beam radiation therapy.

Salvage prostatectomy is more technically challenging than initial radical prostatectomy because of the increased fibrosis and impaired wound healing that follows radiation therapy. Older series have consequently reported high rates of urinary incontinence greater than 70%, bladder neck stricture rates up to 30%, and rectal injury rates of approximately 20%. However, these toxicity rates often improve as centers and surgeons gain more experience with the procedure [Stephenson, Scardino et al. 2004; Nguyen, D'Amico et al. 2007]. The largest reported series of salvage prostatectomy or cystoprostatectomy of 199 patients treated from 1967-2000 at the Mayo Clinic demonstrated improved morbidity rates over time, with incontinence decreasing from 57% to 44% [Ward, Sebo et al. 2005]. Most of these patients had biochemical failure after external beam radiotherapy, although 18 patients were initially treated with brachytherapy as monotherapy and four were initially treated with combined brachytherapy and external beam radiation therapy. Bladder neck contracture was noted in 22% of patients and rectal injury ranged from 5% after prostatectomy alone to 10% after cystoprostatectomy. With a median follow-up of seven years, progression-free survival was 58% at five years and 48% at ten years, although 61% of patients received androgen deprivation therapy after surgery.

Another large series including 100 patients treated with salvage prostatectomy from 1984-2003 at Memorial Sloan-Kettering Cancer Center [Stephenson, Scardino et al. 2004]. Forty two of the patients had local failures after prostate brachytherapy, 28 of which were performed using a retropubic approach and 14 that were performed with a transperineal approach. With a median follow-up of five years after salvage treatment, the five year progression free survival was 55%. Prostate cancer specific survival was 73% at ten years and 60% at 15 years [Bianco, Scardino et al. 2005]. Overall complication rates were worse in patients that had previously been treated with retropubic brachytherapy, and rates of rectal injury and all serious (greater than grade 2) toxicities decreased over time as was observed in the previous series. The overall urinary stricture rate was 30% and was more likely in patients who received prior external beam radiotherapy in comparison to those who were treated with brachytherapy (hazard ratio 4.8, p = 0.04). At five years after salvage, 39% of patients had no evidence of incontinence and 68% used urinary pads less frequently than once daily.

A third large series of 51 patients who underwent salvage prostatectomy from 1983-2002 was reported from the University of Southern California/Norris Cancer Center [Sanderson, Penson et al. 2006], although over half of the patients received androgen deprivation therapy within 30 days of their surgery. Twelve patients were salvaged after they had initially been treated with prostate brachytherapy as monotherapy; eight originally received a combination of external beam therapy and brachytherapy; and one received initial brachytherapy and cryotherapy. Although only 47% of patients remained progression-free at five years (with a median follow-up of 7.2 years), none of patients that had pathologically organ-confined disease at salvage surgery had a biochemical recurrence. Toxicities after salvage surgery included incontinence and bladder neck contractures in more than 40% of patients and rectal injury with subsequent development of a rectourethral fistula in one patient.

Although salvage prostatectomy has typically been performed as an open procedure, options could potentially include robotic and laparoscopic approaches. These types of minimally invasive procedures demonstrated a 67% biochemical relapse-free survival in preliminary reports of a series of 18 patients treated from 2004-2008, although there was a 67% rate of incontinence and a 28% rate of positive margins at the time of surgery [Eandi, Link et al. 2003].

The use of salvage brachytherapy was previously limited because of prior limitations in the dosimetry of initial treatments and the salvage procedures. Consequently, early series reported increased rates of grade 3-4 genitourinary complications and a fistula risk of over 3% [Nguyen, D'Amico et al. 2007]. Incontinence was also commonly noted. Although results have generally improved over time, biochemical relapse-free survival in the largest series reported to date have varied from 30-70% with limited follow up [Grado, Collins et al. 1999; Beyer 2003; Nguyen, D'Amico et al. 2007].

Advancements in the use of dedicated prostate imaging to localize recurrent disease and in brachytherapy's ability to pinpoint the region targeted for retreatment have increased the options available for salvage brachytherapy procedures. It is currently feasible to target the entire gland, the involved lobe or the specific region of recurrence for treatment. Treating smaller areas of the gland will likely lead to decreased toxicity, but it is unknown whether this type of procedure will lead to equivalent disease control. One prospective phase 2 study evaluated the use of MRI-guided salvage brachytherapy performed on 25 men from 2000 - 2005, 11 of whom were initially treated with brachytherapy as monotherapy, and noted a 30% risk of Grade 3 - 4 GI or GU toxicity and a 13% risk of fistulas requiring surgical repair [Nguyen, Chen et al. 2007]. With a median follow-up of 47 months, biochemical relapse-free survival was 70% at 4 years.

Salvage cryotherapy has historically put patients at significant risk for urinary morbidity, although this risk has been ameliorated by recent improvements in the procedure such as use of a transrectal ultrasound guided technique and the utilization of urethral warming catheters. Reported rates of urinary incontinence after the procedure have varied from 30% - 95% [Perrotte, Litwin et al. 1999; Nguyen, D'Amico et al. 2007; Pisters, Rewcastle et al. 2008]. Urethral sloughing, bladder neck stricture, fistulas and perineal pain have also been reported with variable frequency [Perrotte, Litwin et al. 1999; Pisters, Rewcastle et al. 2008] and rates of erectile dysfunction have been high [Touma, Izawa et al. 2005]. Historical series have also often demonstrated decreased efficacy rates for salvage cryotherapy compared with other potential salvage therapies, potentially due to past deficiencies in treating the entire prostate gland or involved region as well as differences in patient selection and definitions of biochemical failure [Izawa, Madsen et al. 2002; Touma, Izawa et al. 2005; Ng, Moussa et al. 2007; Nguyen, D'Amico et al. 2007; Pisters, Rewcastle et al. 2008].

Multi-institutional results were recently reported on 279 patients who underwent salvage cryoablation, 32 of whom were initially treated with brachytherapy as monotherapy and 20 of whom received external beam radiation therapy and a brachytherapy boost [Pisters, Rewcastle et al. 2008]. With a median follow-up of 21.6 months, five-year biochemical relapse-free survival rates was 55-59%, with a 1.2% rate of rectal fistulas and a 4.4% incontinence rate. Impotence was observed in 69% of patients following cryosurgery.

Salvage high-frequency ultrasound is not currently performed in the United States, but has been used in other countries. A series from France demonstrated promising early results in patients who have failed after external beam radiation therapy[Murat, Poissonnier et al. 2009]. The major toxicities noted were related to urination, including urinary sloughing and incontinence. Some patients also developed urethrorectal fistulas after the procedure. Further studies will be needed to further evaluate the effectiveness and morbidity of this salvage option before wider use.

As was true with the studies evaluating the use of prostate brachytherapy as initial treatment for prostate cancer, studies of salvage procedure are also limited by short follow-up, inconsistent definitions of biochemical relapse and the variable use of androgen deprivation therapy[Nguyen, D'Amico et al. 2007; Pisters, Rewcastle et al. 2008]. Future studies will ideally aid in clarifying the patients that are most appropriate candidates for salvage therapy, and which salvage options are most effective. Already, improvements in risk stratification at the time of biochemical failure have helped to identify patients that may derive the most benefit from salvage therapy [Nguyen, D'Amico et al. 2007]. Low Gleason score, decreased PSA velocity and clinical T1c or T2a disease all predict for isolated local recurrence, as does a negative bone scan, negative pelvic imaging and a positive prostate rebiopsy. In our institution, MRI/ultrasound fusion-guided prostate biopsies have been used in select cases to confirm locally recurrent disease in preparation for salvage therapy. Care must be taken as radiation-induced changes can be difficult to interpret on pathology and positive biopsies can take up to 30 months to become negative after initial prostate brachytherapy [Crook, Perry et al. 1995; Stone, Stock et al. 2007]. This is especially of concern given that patients may have a non-significant PSA bounce within the first 24 months after prostate brachytherapy [Horwitz, Levy et al. 2006], which can be misinterpreted as a local failure in the setting of biopsies demonstrating persistent (but likely non-viable) tumor cells that can also occur in this time frame.

Conclusion, Future Directions

In summary, numerous series have demonstrated favorable biochemical relapse-free survival and prostate cancer-specific survival in patients treated with brachytherapy as monotherapy. In low-risk patients, brachytherapy is often the treatment of choice, and the American College of Surgical Oncology Group is currently attempting to conduct a randomized controlled trial to directly evaluate brachytherapy in comparison to radical prostatectomy in patients with favorable risk features (Surgical Prostatectomy versus Interstitial RadiationIntervention Trial – SPIRIT). Although the most favorable results have been demonstrated in patients with low-risk disease, select patients with high-risk disease features may also achieve favorable results after brachytherapy, especially as the ability to select patients with organ-confined cancers improve and with the continued technological improvements that allow for increased treatment precision and dose-escalation. Ongoing clinical trials, such as the current Radiation Therapy Oncology Group (RTOG) Phase II and Phase III trials evaluating the efficacy of prostate brachytherapy alone or in combination with external beam therapy in the treatment of intermediate risk prostate cancer, will attempt to better delineate which patients are appropriate brachytherapy candidates [Lee, DeSilvio et al.

2006]. Indeed, the role of external beam radiation therapy combined with a brachytherapy boost remains undefined, although a number of series have reported favorable outcomes using the two treatments in combination for higher risk patients [Sylvester, Grimm et al. 2001].

In addition to combinations with external beam radiation therapy, brachytherapy is also frequently combined with androgen deprivation therapy. Although the use of androgen deprivation therapy is often limited to short courses intended to reduce the size of enlarged prostates (generally greater than 50 ml) to make them more amenable to brachytherapy, androgen deprivation therapy has also been used for longer periods in patients who have intermediate and high-risk disease. The benefit of androgen deprivation therapy in higher risk and locally advanced disease in combination with external beam therapy has been demonstrated [Bolla, Gonzalez et al. 1997; Denham, Steigler et al. 2005; Horwitz, Bae et al. 2008], but the value of combining androgen deprivation with prostate brachytherapy is unknown.

Local failures within the prostate are rare after brachytherapy, and select patients with local recurrence in the prostate are candidates for local salvage treatments including radical prostatectomy, repeat prostate brachytherapy, cryotherapy or high frequency ultrasound. These treatments have historically been associated with increased toxicity, but technological improvements and growing institutional experiences have led to improved morbidity in more recent series. Although follow-up from these more recent series is limited, salvage procedures have to this point been associated with increased rates of durable local disease control and cure.

Unfortunately, the studies evaluating salvage procedures as well as the overall efficacy of initial treatment with prostate brachytherapy have significant limitations. The lack of randomized controlled trials has limited efficacy data to that largely derived from retrospective series, many of which are single-institution experiences. Thus, comparisons with other treatment modalities are hampered by selection bias even when meticulous attempts are made to control for known prognostic factors. Risk groups are often used to aid in these comparisons, but the criteria for these groups are often incomplete and variable. Additionally, adequate and accurate target delineation and dosimetry clearly impacts efficacy, and older series including suboptimal implants may negatively impact overall results. Finally, because prostate cancer mortality is often delayed by years to decades even with no treatment, biochemical relapse has been used as a surrogate to evaluate the efficacy of prostate cancer treatment. Regrettably, the definition of biochemical relapse has varied with time and is dependent on treatment, although only relatively minor discrepancies in outcomes have been noted in many studies where multiple definitions of biochemical relapse were used in parallel[Thames, Kuban et al. 2003]. Consequently, longer follow up of current and future series will be needed to better determine the effect of prostate brachytherapy on prostate cancer-specific and overall survival[Stock, Cesaretti et al. 2006].

Ongoing technological improvements and innovative concurrent and adjuvant therapies will likely further increase the efficacy of prostate brachytherapy. Although LDR treatments have been most frequently performed in the United States, HDR treatments have also demonstrated promise either alone or in combination with external beam radiation therapy[Hoskin 2000; Grills, Martinez et al. 2004; Yoshioka, Konishi et al. 2006; Pisansky, Gold et al. 2008]. Whether an increased dose rate will lead to greater durable long-term disease control is unknown. Current prostate brachytherapy planning is typically performed with the aid of transrectal ultrasound imaging, but CT and even MRI guided brachytherapy has been investigated [D'Amico, Cormack et al. 1998]. Future imaging improvements could even facilitate combining prostate brachytherapy with functional prostate cancer imaging to allow more precise targeting of diseased areas of the gland. Finally, brachytherapy has already been used in combination with external beam radiation therapy and androgen deprivation therapy, but whether these treatments increase cure rates and in which subgroups of patients they are efficacious remain unknown. Patients with multiple high risk features, e.g. higher Gleason score, high pretreatment-PSA, among others, are more likely to fail distally with metastatic disease after any initial prostate cancer treatment including brachytherapy and are, therefore, good candidates for these investigational approaches.

References

Bagshaw, M. A., Kaplan, I. D. et al. (1993). "Prostate cancer. Radiation therapy for localized disease." *Cancer, 71(3 Suppl)*, 939-52.

Barringer, B. S. (1924). "RADIUM IN THE TREATMENT OF PROSTATIC CARCINOMA." *Ann Surg, 80(6)*, 881-4.

Barringer, B. S. (1938). "Radiotherapy of Tumors of the Urinary Tract." *Bull N Y Acad Med, 14(5)*, 252-8.

Battermann, J. J., Boon, T. A. et al. (2004). "Results of permanent prostate brachytherapy, 13 years of experience at a single institution." Radiotherapy and oncology: *journal of the European Society for Therapeutic Radiology and Oncology, 71(1)*, 23-8.

Beard, C., Schultz, D. et al. (2006). "Perineural invasion associated with increased cancer-specific mortality after external beam radiation therapy for men with low- and intermediate-risk prostate cancer." *Int J Radiat Oncol Biol Phys., 66(2)*, 403-7.

Beyer, D. C. (2003). "Brachytherapy for recurrent prostate cancer after radiation therapy." *SeminRadiatOncol, 13(2)*, 158-65.

Beyer, D. C., Brachman, D. G. (2000). "Failure free survival following brachytherapy alone for prostate cancer: comparison with external beam radiotherapy." Radiotherapy and oncology: *journal of the European Society for Therapeutic Radiology and Oncology, 57(3)*, 263-7.

Bianco, F. J., Scardino, P. T. et al. (2005). "Long-term oncologic results of salvage radical prostatectomy for locally recurrent prostate cancer after radiotherapy." *Int J Radiat Oncol Biol Phys., 62(2)*, 448-53.

Bill-Axelson, A., Holmberg, L. et al. (2008). "Radical prostatectomy versus watchful waiting in localized prostate cancer: the Scandinavian prostate cancer group-4 randomized trial." *J Natl Cancer Inst., 100(16)*, 1144-54.

Block, T., Czempiel, H. et al. (2006). "Transperineal permanent seed implantation of "low-risk" prostate cancer: 5-year-experiences in 118 patients." *Strahlenther Onkol, 182(11)*, 666-71.

Bolla, M., Gonzalez, D. et al. (1997). "Improved survival in patients with locally advanced prostate cancer treated with radiotherapy and goserelin." *N Engl J Med, 337(5)*, 295-300.

Brachman, D. G., Thomas, T. et al. (2000). "Failure-free survival following brachytherapy alone or external beam irradiation alone for T1-2 prostate tumors in 2222 patients: results from a single practice." *IntJRadiatOncolBiolPhys., 48(1)*, 111-7.

Buron, C., Le Vu, B. et al. (2007). "Brachytherapy versus prostatectomy in localized prostate cancer: results of a French multicenter prospective medico-economic study." *Int J Radiat Oncol Biol Phys.*, *67(3)*, 812-22.

Chong, C. C. W., Austen, L. et al. (2006). "Patterns of practice in the management of prostate cancer: results from multidisciplinary surveys of clinicians in Australia and New Zealand in 1995 and 2000." *BJU Int.*, *97(5)*, 975-80.

Cooperberg, M. R., Grossfeld, G. D. et al. (2003). "National practice patterns and time trends in androgen ablation for localized prostate cancer." *J Natl Cancer Inst.*, *95(13)*, 981-9.

Cooperberg, M. R., Moul, J. W. et al. (2005). "The changing face of prostate cancer." *J Clin Oncol, 23(32)*, 8146-51.

Crook, J. M., Perry, G. A. et al. (1995). "Routine prostate biopsies following radiotherapy for prostate cancer: results for 226 patients." *Urology, 45(4)*, 624-31; discussion 631-2.

D'Amico, A. V., Cormack, R. et al. (1998). "Real-time magnetic resonance image-guided interstitial brachytherapy in the treatment of select patients with clinically localized prostate cancer." *Int J Radiat Oncol Biol Phys.*, *42(3)*, 507-15.

D'Amico, A. V., Renshaw, A. A., et al. (2004). "Impact of the percentage of positive prostate cores on prostate cancer-specific mortality for patients with low or favorable intermediate-risk disease." *J Clin Oncol, 22(18)*, 3726-32.

D'Amico, A. V., Renshaw, A. A., et al. (2005). "Pretreatment PSA velocity and risk of death from prostate cancer following external beam radiation therapy." *JAMA, 294(4)*, 440-7.

D'Amico, A. V., Whittington, R., et al. (1998). "Biochemical outcome after radical prostatectomy, external beam radiation therapy, or interstitial radiation therapy for clinically localized prostate cancer." *JAMA, 280(11)*, 969-74.

D'Amico, A. V., Whittington, R., et al. (1996). "Critical analysis of the ability of the endorectal coil magnetic resonance imaging scan to predict pathologic stage, margin status, and postoperative prostate-specific antigen failure in patients with clinically organ-confined prostate cancer." *J Clin Oncol, 14(6)*, 1770-7.

Denham, J. W., Steigler, A., et al. (2005). "Short-term androgen deprivation and radiotherapy for locally advanced prostate cancer: results from the Trans-Tasman Radiation Oncology Group 96.01 randomised controlled trial." *LancetOncol, 6(11)*, 841-50.

Eandi, J. A., Link, B. A., et al. (2003). "Robotic Assisted Laparoscopic Salvage Prostatectomy for Radiation Resistant Prostate Cancer." *JURO, 1-5*.

Grado, G. L., Collins, J. M., et al. (1999). "Salvage brachytherapy for localized prostate cancer after radiotherapy failure." *Urology, 53(1)*, 2-10.

Grills, I. S., Martinez, A. A. et al. (2004). "High dose rate brachytherapy as prostate cancer monotherapy reduces toxicity compared to low dose rate palladium seeds." *TheJournalofUrology, 171(3)*, 1098-104.

Grimm, P. D., Blasko, J. C., et al. (2001). "10-year biochemical (prostate-specific antigen) control of prostate cancer with (125)I brachytherapy." *Int J Radiat Oncol Biol Phys.*, *51(1)*, 31-40.

Guedea, F., Aguilo, F., et al. (2006). "Early biochemical outcomes following permanent interstitial brachytherapy as monotherapy in 1050 patients with clinical T1-T2 prostate cancer." Radiotherapy and oncology: *journaloftheEuropeanSocietyfor Therapeuti cRadiologyandOncology, 80(1)*, 57-61.

Guedea, F., Ellison, T., et al. (2007). "Overview of brachytherapy resources in Europe: a survey of patterns of care study for brachytherapy in Europe." Radiotherapy and oncology: *journal of the European Society for Therapeutic Radiology and Oncology, 82(1)*, 50-4.

Henry, A. M., Al-Qaisieh, B., et al. (2010). "Outcomes following iodine-125 monotherapy for localized prostate cancer: the results of leeds 10-year single-center brachytherapy experience." *IntJRadiatOncolBiolPhys., 76(1)*, 50-6.

Hinnen, K. A., Battermann, J. J., et al. (2009). "Long-Term Biochemical and Survival Outcome of 921 Patients Treated with I-125 Permanent Prostate Brachytherapy." *IntJRadiatOncolBiolPhys.*

Holm, H. H. (1997). "The history of interstitial brachytherapy of prostatic cancer." *SeminSurgOncol, 13(6)*, 431-7.

Horwitz, E. M., Bae, K., et al. (2008). "Ten-year follow-up of radiation therapy oncology group protocol 92-02: a phase III trial of the duration of elective androgen deprivation in locally advanced prostate cancer." *JClinOncol, 26(15)*, 2497-504.

Horwitz, E. M., Levy, L. B., et al. (2006). "Biochemical and clinical significance of the posttreatment prostate-specific antigen bounce for prostate cancer patients treated with external beam radiation therapy alone: a multiinstitutional pooled analysis." *Cancer, 107(7)*, 1496-502.

Hoskin, P. J. (2000). "High dose rate brachytherapy boost treatment in radical radiotherapy for prostate cancer." Radiotherapy and oncology: *journaloftheEuropeanSoci etyforTherapeuticRadiologyandOncology, 57(3)*, 285-8.

Izawa, J. I., Madsen, L. T., et al. (2002). "Salvage cryotherapy for recurrent prostate cancer after radiotherapy: variables affecting patient outcome." *J Clin Oncol, 20(11)*, 2664-71.

Kao, J., Stone, N. N., et al. (2008). "(125)I monotherapy using D90 implant doses of 180 Gy or greater." *IntJRadiatOncolBiolPhys., 70(1)*, 96-101.

Kattan, M. W., Stapleton, A. M., et al. (1997). "Evaluation of a nomogram used to predict the pathologic stage of clinically localized prostate carcinoma." *Cancer, 79(3)*, 528-37.

Klein, E. A., Ciezki, J., et al. (2008). "Outcomes for intermediate risk prostate cancer: Are there advantages for surgery, external radiation, or brachytherapy?" *Urol Oncol, 27(1)*, 67-71.

Kollmeier, M. A., Stock, R. G., et al. (2003). "Biochemical outcomes after prostate brachytherapy with 5-year minimal follow-up: importance of patient selection and implant quality." *Int J Radiat Oncol Biol Phys., 57(3)*, 645-53.

Kuban, D. A., Levy, L. B., et al. (2006). "Comparison of biochemical failure definitions for permanent prostate brachytherapy." *Int J Radiat Oncol Biol Phys., 65(5)*, 1487-93.

Kupelian, P. A., Potters, L. et al. (2004). "Radical prostatectomy, external beam radiotherapy<72 Gy, external beam radiotherapy > or =72 Gy, permanent seed implantation, or combined seeds/external beam radiotherapy for stage T1-T2 prostate cancer." *Int J Radiat Oncol Biol Phys., 58(1)*, 25-33.

Lawrentschuk, N., Fleshner, N. (2009). "The role of magnetic resonance imaging in targeting prostate cancer in patients with previous negative biopsies and elevated prostate-specific antigen levels." *BJU International, 103(6)*, 730-3.

Lee, W. R., DeSilvio, M., et al. (2006). "A phase II study of external beam radiotherapy combined with permanent source brachytherapy for intermediate-risk, clinically localized adenocarcinoma of the prostate: preliminary results of RTOG P-0019." *IntJRadiat OncolBiolPhys., 64(3)*, 804-9.

Lieberfarb, M. E., Schultz, D., et al. (2002). "Using PSA, biopsy Gleason score, clinical stage, and the percentage of positive biopsies to identify optimal candidates for prostate-only radiation therapy." *Int J Radiat Oncol Biol Phys.*, *53(4)*, 898-903.

Merrick, G. S., Butler, W. M., et al. (2004). "Permanent interstitial brachytherapy in younger patients with clinically organ-confined prostate cancer." *Urology*, *64(4)*, 754-9.

Merrick, G. S., Butler, W. M., et al. (2005). "Impact of supplemental external beam radiotherapy and/or androgen deprivation therapy on biochemical outcome after permanent prostate brachytherapy." *Int J Radiat Oncol Biol Phys.*, *61(1)*, 32-43.

Merrick, G. S., Wallner, K. E., et al. (2006). "Brachytherapy in men aged < or = 54 years with clinically localized prostate cancer." *BJU Int.*, *98(2)*, 324-8.

Merrick, G. S., Wallner, K. E., et al. (2008). "Prostate brachytherapy in men > or =75 years of age." *IntJRadiatOncolBiolPhys.*, *72(2)*, 415-20.

Mitchell, D. M., Mandall, P., et al. (2008). "Report on the Early Efficacy and Tolerability of I125 Permanent Prostate Brachytherapy from a UK Multi-institutional Database." *Clinical Oncology*, *20(10)*, 738-744.

Morris, W. J., Keyes, M., et al. (2009). "Population-based study of biochemical and survival outcomes after permanent 125I brachytherapy for low- and intermediate-risk prostate cancer." *Urology*, *73(4)*, 860-5, discussion 865-7.

Murat, F. J., Poissonnier, L., et al. (2009). "Mid-term results demonstrate salvage high-intensity focused ultrasound (HIFU) as an effective and acceptably morbid salvage treatment option for locally radiorecurrent prostate cancer." *Eur Urol*, *55(3)*, 640-7.

Nag, S., Bice, W., et al. (2000). "The American Brachytherapy Society recommendations for permanent prostate brachytherapy postimplant dosimetric analysis." *Int J Radiat Oncol Biol Phys.*, *46(1)*, 221-30.

National Comprehensive Cancer Network, T. N. C. C. (2009). "NCCN Practice Guidelines in Oncology - Prostate Cancer." *NCCN Clinical Practice Guidelines in Oncology*, v.2. 2009, 1-46.

Ng, C. K., Moussa, M., et al. (2007). "Salvage cryoablation of the prostate: followup and analysis of predictive factors for outcome." *TheJournalofUrology*, *178(4 Pt 1)*, 1253-7; discussion 1257.

Nguyen, P. L., Chen, M. H., et al. (2007). "Magnetic resonance image-guided salvage brachytherapy after radiation in select men who initially presented with favorable-risk prostate cancer: a prospective phase 2 study." *Cancer*, *110(7)*, 1485-92.

Nguyen, P. L., D'Amico, A. V., et al. (2007). "Patient selection, cancer control, and complications after salvage local therapy for postradiation prostate-specific antigen failure: a systematic review of the literature." *Cancer*, *110(7)*, 1417-28.

Partin, A. W., Mangold, L. A., et al. (2001). "Contemporary update of prostate cancer staging nomograms (Partin Tables) for the new millennium." *Urology*, *58(6)*, 843-8.

Perrotte, P., Litwin, M. S., et al. (1999). "Quality of life after salvage cryotherapy: the impact of treatment parameters." *TheJournalofUrology*, *162(2)*, 398-402.

Pisansky, T. M., Gold, D. G., et al. (2008). "High-dose-rate brachytherapy in the curative treatment of patients with localized prostate cancer." *MayoClinProc.*, *83(12)*, 1364-72.

Pisters, L. L., Rewcastle, J. C., et al. (2008). "Salvage prostate cryoablation: initial results from the cryo on-line data registry." *TheJournalofUrology*, *180(2)*, 559-63; discussion 563-4.

Polascik, T. J., Pound, C. R., et al. (1998). "Comparison of radical prostatectomy and iodine 125 interstitial radiotherapy for the treatment of clinically localized prostate cancer: a 7-year biochemical (PSA) progression analysis." *Urology, 51(6)*, 884-9; discussion 889-90.

Potosky, A. L., Miller, B. A., et al. (1995). "The role of increasing detection in the rising incidence of prostate cancer." *JAMA, 273(7)*, 548-52.

Potters, L., Morgenstern, C., et al. (2005). "12-year outcomes following permanent prostate brachytherapy in patients with clinically localized prostate cancer." *TheJourna lofUrology, 173(5)*, 1562-6.

Pound, C. R., Partin, A. W., et al. (1999). "Natural history of progression after PSA elevation following radical prostatectomy." *JAMA, 281(17)*, 1591-7.

Ragde, H., Korb, L. J., et al. (2000). "Modern prostate brachytherapy. Prostate specific antigen results in 219 patients with up to 12 years of observed follow-up." *Cancer, 89(1)*, 135-41.

Ramos, C. G., Carvalhal, G. F., et al. (1999). "Retrospective comparison of radical retropubic prostatectomy and 125iodine brachytherapy for localized prostate cancer." *The Journal ofUrology, 161(4)*, 1212-5.

Roach, M., Hanks, G., et al. (2006). "Defining biochemical failure following radiotherapy with or without hormonal therapy in men with clinically localized prostate cancer: recommendations of the RTOG-ASTRO Phoenix Consensus Conference." *IntJRadiatOncolBiolPhys., 65(4)*, 965-74.

Sanda, M. G., Dunn, R. L., et al. (2008). "Quality of life and satisfaction with outcome among prostate-cancer survivors." *N Engl J Med, 358(12)*, 1250-61.

Sanderson, K. M., Penson, D. F., et al. (2006). "Salvage radical prostatectomy: quality of life outcomes and long-term oncological control of radiorecurrent prostate cancer." *TheJournalofUrology, 176(5)*, 2025-31; discussion 2031-2.

Stephenson, A. J., Scardino, P. T., et al. (2004). "Morbidity and functional outcomes of salvage radical prostatectomy for locally recurrent prostate cancer after radiation therapy." *TheJournalofUrology, 172(6 Pt 1)*, 2239-43.

Stock, R. G., Cesaretti, J. A., et al. (2006). "Disease-specific survival following the brachytherapymanagement of prostate cancer." *IntJRadiatOncolBiolPhys., 64(3)*, 810-6.

Stock, R. G., Stone, N. N. et al. (1998). "A dose-response study for I-125 prostate implants." *Int J Radiat Oncol Biol Phys., 41(1)*, 101-8.

Stone, N. N., Potters, L., et al. (2007). "Customized dose prescription for permanent prostate brachytherapy: insights from a multicenter analysis of dosimetry outcomes." *IntJRadiatOncolBiolPhys., 69(5)*, 1472-7.

Stone, N. N., Stock, R. G., et al. (2009). "Local Control Following Permanent Prostate Brachytherapy: Effect of High Biologically Effective Dose on Biopsy Results and Oncologic Outcomes." *IntJRadiatOncolBiolPhys.*

Stone, N. N., Stock, R. G., et al. (2005). "Intermediate term biochemical-free progression and local control following 125iodine brachytherapy for prostate cancer." *TheJournalofUrology, 173(3)*, 803-7.

Stone, N. N., Stock, R. G., et al. (2007). "Patterns of local failure following prostate brachytherapy." *The Journal of Urology, 177(5)*, 1759-63, duscussion 1763-4.

Sylvester, J., Grimm, P., et al. (2001). "The role of androgen ablation in patients with biochemical or local failure after definitive radiation therapy: a survey of practice patterns of urologists and radiation oncologists in the United States." *Urology, 58(2 Suppl 1)*, 65-70.

Taira, A. V., Merrick, G. S., et al. (2009). "Natural History of Clinically Staged Low- and Intermediate-Risk Prostate Cancer Treated With Monotherapeutic Permanent Interstitial Brachytherapy." *IntJRadiatOncolBiolPhys*.

Thames, H., Kuban, D., et al. (2003). "Comparison of alternative biochemical failure definitions based on clinical outcome in 4839 prostate cancer patients treated by external beam radiotherapy between 1986 and 1995." *IntJRadiatOncolBiolPhys, 57(4)*, 929-43.

Touma, N. J., Izawa, J. I., et al. (2005). "Current status of local salvage therapies following radiation failure for prostate cancer." *TheJournalofUrology, 173(2)*, 373-9.

Turkbey, B., Pinto, P. A., et al. (2009). "Imaging techniques for prostate cancer: implications for focal therapy." *NatRevUrol., 6(4)*, 191-203.

Wallner, K., Merrick, G., et al. (2005). "High-dose regions versus likelihood of cure after prostate brachytherapy." *IntJRadiatOncolBiolPhys., 62(1)*, 170-4.

Wallner, K., Merrick, G., et al. (2003). "125I versus 103Pd for low-risk prostate cancer: preliminary PSA outcomes from a prospective randomized multicenter trial." *IntJRadiatOncolBiolPhys., 57(5)*, 1297-303.

Ward, J. F., Sebo, T. J., et al. (2005). "Salvage surgery for radiorecurrent prostate cancer: contemporary outcomes." *The Journal of Urology, 173(4)*, 1156-60.

Whitmore, W. F., Hilaris, B., et. al. (1972). "Retropubic implantation to iodine-125 in the treatment of prostatic cancer." *TheJournalofUrology, 108(6)*, 918-20.

Yoshioka, Y. (2009). "Current status and perspectives of brachytherapy for prostate cancer." *Int J Clin Oncol, 14(1)*, 31-6.

Yoshioka, Y., Konishi, K., et al. (2006). "High-dose-rate brachytherapy without external beam irradiation for locally advanced prostate cancer." Radiotherapy and oncology: *journaloftheEuropeanSocietyforTherapeuticRadiologyandOncology, 80(1)*, 62-8.

Zelefsky, M. J., Kuban, D. A., et al. (2007). "Multi-institutional analysis of long-term outcome for stages T1-T2 prostate cancer treated with permanent seed implantation." *Int J Radiat Oncol Biol Phys., 67(2)*, 327-33.

Zelefsky, M. J., Yamada, Y., et al. (2000). "Postimplantation dosimetric analysis of permanent transperineal prostate implantation: improved dose distributions with an intraoperative computer-optimized conformal planning technique." *Int J Radiat Oncol Biol Phys., 48(2)*, 601-8.

Zelefsky, M. J., Yamada, Y., et al. (2007). "Five-year outcome of intraoperative conformal permanent I-125 interstitial implantation for patients with clinically localized prostate cancer." *Int J Radiat Oncol Biol Phys., 67(1)*, 65-70.

In: Brachytherapy
Editor: Leoni M. Fischer

ISBN: 978-1-61728-750-3
© 2011 Nova Science Publishers, Inc.

Chapter 2

High-Dose-Rate Interstitial Brachytherapy in the Management of Primary and Recurrent Gynaecologic Malignancies: Clinical Experience and Review of the Literature

Isabelle Thibault and Eric Vigneault[*]
Département de Radio-oncologie, L'Hôtel-Dieu de Québec, Centre Hospitalier
Universitaire de Québec (CHUQ), Québec, QC, Canada

Abstract

Purpose: To evaluate the outcomes, toxicities and dose-volume histogram (DVH) parameters of high-dose-rate interstitial brachytherapy (HDR-ISBT) in the management of primary and recurrent gynaecologic malignancies.

Materials and Methods: Between 2001 and 2009, 38 patients with gynaecologic cancer were treated at L'Hotel-Dieu de Quebec with Ir-192 remote afterloading HDR-ISBT, using a Syed-Neblett template for implant technique and inverse planning simulated annealing (IPSA) algorithm for dosimetry optimization. The median HDR-ISBT dose delivered was 30Gy (range: 18–35), given in 4–6 Gy/fraction. All patients received pelvic external beam radiation therapy (EBRT). Four patients with vaginal recurrence (R) also had previous intracavitary brachytherapy (ICBT). Toxicities were assessed according to CTCAE v3.0. Total equivalent dose in 2-Gy fractions (EQD$_2$) was calculated, combining HDR-ISBT and EBRT contributions. Results were compared with published data.

Results: Of the 38 patients reviewed, 30 were treated for primary malignancies (PM) of the vagina (n=15), cervix (n=9), vulva (n=2) or Bartholin's gland (n=4) and 8 had recurrent gynaecologic cancer. FIGO stage distribution for PM was: I (n=2), II (n=12), III

[*] Corresponding author: Email: Eric.Vigneault@chuq.qc.ca, Département de Radio-oncologie, CHUQ-HDQ, 11 Côte du Palais, Québec (Québec), Canada, G1R 2J6; Tel: 418 691-5264; Fax : 418 691-5268.

(n=13), IV (n=3). Median age was 57. Median follow-up was 20.6 months (range: 1-92). Complete response rate (CR) was 82% for PM versus 75% for R. Local control (LC) for PM and R was 86.7 vs 37.5% at 2 years and 81.3 vs. 37.5% at 5 years (p=0.007). 5-year overall survival was 78.9 vs 14.3% (p<0.001). DVH parameters for target volume showed a median V100 of 97.5% and EQD$_2$ D90 and D100 of 89Gy$_{10}$ and 69Gy$_{10}$. For OAR, median dose to 2cc (D$_{2cc}$) was 80.1Gy$_3$ for rectum and 76.9Gy$_3$ for bladder. These DVH values appear to be at least equivalent to those published for MRI guided ICBT following the GEC-ESTRO recommendations, except for our rectal D$_{2cc}$ that was higher. The median D$_{0.1cc}$ for urethra was 79.7Gy$_3$. Twelve patients experienced grade 3-4 late toxicities (gastrointestinal and genitourinary) but only two of them were still suffering from grade 3-4 toxicity at last follow-up.

Conclusion: The use of HDR-ISBT offers good long-term LC, especially in PM, at a cost of possible transitory severe late toxicities. This therapeutic option should be considered for PM that cannot be optimally treated with ICBT and for isolated R. DVH parameters of OARs recommended by the Gyn GEC-ESTRO and urethral D0.1cc or D10 should be reported. Further investigations are needed to define dose-volume constraints in HDR-ISBT.

Introduction

Brachytherapy has become an integral component of the therapeutic management of gynaecologic cancers in the last century. A standard combination in the treatment algorithm is the use of external beam radiation therapy (EBRT) followed by brachytherapy. EBRT is delivered first to reduce the tumoral bulk and to facilitate brachytherapy. A higher dose to the target is achieved with brachytherapy to improve local control while sparing the surrounding normal organs from radiation. Traditionally, an intracavitary system was used, consisting of an intrauterine tandem and two vaginal ovoid applicators. Treatment planning was based on a two-dimensional (2D) imaging. Orthogonal radiographs were obtained and dose was calculated at point A and point B, derived from the classical Manchester system [1]. Estimates of doses to organs at risk (OARs) were subsequently recorded such as the dose at the bladder and rectal reference points, defined by the International Commission on Radiation Units (ICRU) report 38 [2].

Since the 1990s, advances in three-dimensional (3D) imaging technology, such as computed tomography (CT) and magnetic resonance imaging (MRI), have enabled more precise delineation of target volumes and critical organs for radiotherapy planning in patients with gynaecologic malignancies [3]. The Groupe Européen de Curiethérapie and the European Society for Therapeutic Radiology and Oncology (GEC-ESTRO) have recently formulated recommendations to advocate 3D image-based treatment planning for intracavitary brachytherapy, with emphasis on MRI-based planning [4]. The American Brachytherapy Society (ABS) agreed to adopt these guidelines in 2005 [3]. From the traditional approach using 2D-imaging and point dose assessment, the current practice in intracavitary brachytherapy is slowly integrating 3D computerized planning, prescription of dose to a target volume and the use of dose-volume histogram (DVH) analysis for the OARs.

When a tumor cannot be optimally encompassed by intracavitary brachytherapy, interstitial brachytherapy is preferred, to improve tumor coverage and dose distribution [5-6]. Low-dose-rate (LDR) technique was typically employed until high-dose rate (HDR) interstitial brachytherapy (ISBT) emerged about 20 years ago. The interest in HDR-ISBT has grown since then, mainly because of its potential advantages based on radiobiological, technical and practical considerations. These advantages include the possibility of a superior clinical efficacy, an individualized treatment with source optimization, immobilization of the target, accuracy of source positioning, shorter treatment time, less patient discomfort, possibility of outpatient treatment procedure and complete radioprotection for health care personnel [7-10]. However, an important concern for HDR-ISBT is the risk of acute and late complications in normal tissues. Even though HDR-ISBT has been used in many centers in North America and worldwide, there are very few clinical data regarding this technique compared with LDR-ISBT or with conventional intracavitary brachytherapy. Furthermore, literature is lacking on 3D dose optimization using CT or MRI for gynaecological HDR-ISBT.

The aim of this chapter is to evaluate the pattern of use, the clinical outcomes and the DVH parameters of CT-based HDR-ISBT in women with primary and recurrent gynaecologic malignancies and to review the published literature.

Materials and Methods

Study Population

Between March 2001 and August 2009, 40 patients were treated with gynaecological HDR Iridium-192 ISBT at l'Hôtel-Dieu de Québec using inverse planning. Patient eligibility for interstitial brachytherapy was assessed according to the ABS recommendations[5-6]. The Karnofsky performance status score was 70 or higher in all patients. From this cohort, two patients were excluded because they had vaginal recurrence of non-gynaecologic (rectal) cancer. The 38 patients who remained had primary (n=30) or recurrent (n=8) gynaecologic malignancies, confirmed by biopsy. All patients underwent a complete work-up before treatment and staging was recorded according to the International Federation of Gynaecology and Oncology (FIGO) classification in effect at that time in our institution. The revised FIGO staging published in 2009 was not yet in use. We present in this chapter this retrospective study conducted in 38 patients.

External Beam Radiotherapy and Prior Treatment

All patients received pelvic EBRT, either as part of the standard combined treatment of EBRT and brachytherapy (n=33) or either previously in 5 women affected by a recurrence. Four patients of our sample treated with HDR-ISBT for a recurrent tumoralso had past intracavitary brachytherapy, administered by LDR or HDR.

Brachytherapy Procedure and Treatment Planning

The implantation procedure consisted of catheter insertion through a Syed-Neblett gynaecologic template (Best Medical International Inc., Springfield, VA). The technique was previously described in details for LDR-ISBT [11-15]. It was performed under general anesthesia in the operating room. Gold seed markers were first implanted for identification of tumor position. An intrauterine tandem applicator was inserted in 14 patients, with or without the use of a Hegar's dilator. The plastic vaginal cylinder was placed over the tandem and the perineal template was threaded over the vaginal guide. Either fluoroscopy or transrectal ultrasound was used to guide the needle placement. Moreover, since 2009, MR images are obtained in order to evaluate the high risk clinical target volume (HR-CTV). After insertion, the template was sutured at its four corners to the perineal skin. A post-impant flexible cystoscopy was done to ensure the bladder and the urethra were not perforated and a Foley catheter was placed in the bladder. All patients underwent a single implant and had a lumbar epidural catheter for pain control in the post-operative recovery period and over the duration of the brachytherapy fractionated treatment.

After the procedure, a CT scan was obtained to verify the proper positioning of the catheters and for treatment planning purpose. The clinical target volume (CTV) and OARs including rectum, bladder, urethra and bowel were contoured using PLATO treatment planning system (Nucletron BV, The Netherlands). Dosimetry optimization was performed using the inverse planning simulated annealing (IPSA) algorithm[16]. Dose constraints were adjusted to maximize the target coverage, while minimizing the dose to OARs. The first aim was to achieve a percentage of the CTV receiving 100% of the prescribed dose (V100) exceeding 95%. Figure 1 shows an example of dosimetry. The first treatment was delivered the same day immediately after the planning, using microSelectron HDR remote afterloading system as shown in Figure 2. Subsequent fractions were given twice daily, with a minimum interval of 6 hours between fractions. The median number of catheters used to deliver the radiation was 17 (range: 7–35). Patients received a median total dose of 30 Gy (range: 18–35) by HDR-ISBT, given in 4-6 Gy per fraction.

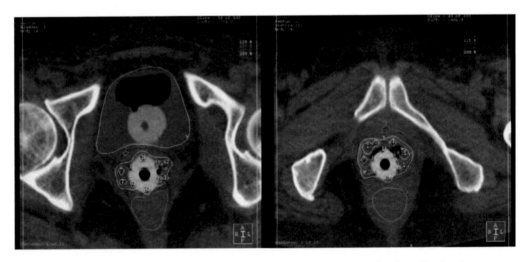

Figure 1. Computed tomography-based interstitial implant using IPSA and isodose distribution on two different axial images. One hundred percent isodose line is in red, 75% in green, 125% in yellow, 150% in light blue, 175% in blue and 200% in white.

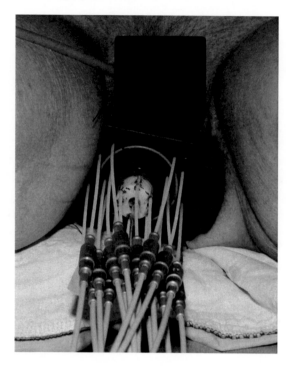

Figure 2. Photograph of a gynaecologic interstitial implant. The gynaecologic template (purple) is fixed to the perineum with the vaginal obturator in place. The 30-cm flexible catheters are marked for position and connected to the transfer tubes of the remote afterloading HDR Ir-192 unit.

DVH analysis

DVH analysis was conducted retrospectively and parameters were reported according to the Gynaecological (Gyn) GEC-ESTRO Working Group [4, 17]. Our definition of the CTV for uterine cervical cancer was in good accordance to the HR-CTV defined by the Gyn GEC-ESTRO. As for the delineation of OARs, only the whole organs (outer wall) were contoured and the sigmoid was not delineated. The DVH was generated using 100,000 sampling points. The minimum dose delivered to 90% and 100% of the CTV (D90, D100), the V100, the volume in cubic centimetres (cc) receiving 150% and 200% of the prescribed dose (V150, V200) and the minimum dose to the most irradiated 0.1, 1 and 2 cc volume ($D_{0.1cc}$, D_{1cc}, and D_{2cc} respectively) of the rectum and bladder were calculated. Urethra DVH parameters $D_{0.1cc}$ and D10 were computed. Homogeneity index (HI) was recorded in all plans to assess the volume of the hot spots relative to the treated volume[18]. HI is defined as:

$$HI = 1 - \left(\frac{V150}{V100}\right)$$

Doses were converted to biologically equivalent dose in 2-Gy fractions (EQD_2) using the linear quadratic model, with α/β ratio of 10 for tumorand α/β of 3 for late effects in normal tissues. The total radiation doses were evaluated in terms of EQD_2, combining contributions from EBRT and HDR-ISBT. It was assumed that the target volume and OARs received the full dose of EBRT. The following formulas were used:

$$EQD_2 = nd \, \frac{(d + \alpha/\beta)}{(2 + \alpha/\beta)}$$

$$EQD_{2\,Total} = EQD_{2\,EBRT} + EQD_{2\,HDR-ISBT}$$

where n was the number of fractions delivered and d was the dose per fraction.

For four patients, past history of orthogonal film-based intracavitary brachytherapy raises the issues of assessing and calculating the corresponding total dose received. In order to adequately evaluate the cumulative dose received in normal tissues for late effects, adding intracavitary contribution to the total EQD_2 dose was required. Because two of the four patients underwent an extensive salvage surgery between the combined EBRT – intracavitary brachytherapy treatment and HDR-ISBT, we assumed that some irradiated tissues were resected. Therefore, we couldn't calculate the total dose to OARs for them. These two women were censored in the DVH analysis. The DVH parameters of HDR-ISBT were unavailable for a third patient. EQD_2 doses of intracavitary brachytherapy were added to the cumulative EQD_2 sum of the fourth patient for evaluation of late effects. She received 24 Gy in 4 fractions by HDR intracavitary brachytherapy. A dose modifying factor (DMF) of 0.7 was applied to the estimation of intracavitary dose contribution in OARs, to account for the fall-off in dose with distance and to calculate a more realistic normal tissue effect [19], as follows.

$$EQD_{2\,Intravacitary} = \frac{nd*DMF*\left(1 + \frac{d*DMF}{\alpha/\beta}\right)}{\left(1 + \frac{2}{\alpha/\beta}\right)}$$

Outcome Assessment

After treatment, patients were followed every 1-3 months for the first 6 months, every 3-6 months for the next 2 years and at 6- to 12-month intervals thereafter. The principal radiation oncologist who performed the implant provided the follow-up visits. A gynaecologic oncologist followed also the patients in a majority of cases. The response to treatment was assessed according to the RECIST criteria. Local failure was defined as disease progression to vagina, cervix or parametria. All local recurrences were biopsy-proven. Regional recurrence was defined as evidence of tumor within the pelvis. Para-aortic lymph node metastases were considered a distant failure. Time to recurrence and survival were calculated from the completion of HDR-ISBT to the date of the event or to the last follow-up. Acute and late toxicities were graded according to the National Cancer Institute Common Terminology Criteria for Adverse Events (NCI CTCAE, version 3.0), considering the worst grade documented. Acute morbidity was defined as symptoms experienced during the course of HDR-ISBT and up to 90 days after.

Statistical Methods

Categorical variables were presented for primary and recurrent gynaecologic malignancies. Quantitative non-normally distributed variables were reported as median and interquartile range (IQR) and categorical variables as numbers and percentages. The following four end points were analyzed: local control, disease-free survival, overall survival and disease-specific survival. Survival curves were constructed using the Kaplan-Meier method and the log-rank test was used to assess differences between groups.

The association between the response to treatment, the occurrence of a local recurrence or the occurrence of toxicity and various clinical and demographics categorical variables were explored in univariate analysis, using univariate exact logistic regression models. Due to small sample size and frequencies of binary events, exact logistic regression modeling based on permutation resampling for estimating the parameters of the logistic models, were utilized. In contrast to standard asymptotic logistic regression methods, which assume sufficiently large sample sizes, exact logistic regression is a conservative approach that remains valid and gives reliable answers for analyzing small, skewed, unbalanced or sparse data sets. The continuous variables were dichotomized based on conventional cut-off values. The logistic regression results are presented as exact odds ratios (OR) with exact 95% confidence interval (CI) and exact p-values.

All statistical analyses were performed using SAS 9.2 software (SAS Institute, Cary, NC). All p-values are two-sided and a p-value < 0.05 was considered statistically significant.

Results

Patient and Tumor Characteristics

The demographic and clinical characteristics of the study population are presented in Table 1. A total of 38 patients underwent 3D image-based HDR-ISBT and were reviewed. The median age of the cohort at the time of the brachytherapy procedure was 56.5 years (range: 34-82 years). The most prevalent comorbid conditions were: current smoking (21%), hypertension (29%), coronary artery disease (11%) and obesity (11%). Fourteen and nineteen patients had respectively a previous hysterectomy for a benign disease or a previous abdominal or pelvic surgery before the diagnosis of gynaecological malignancy. Six patients had also a past medical history of cancer, including cervical carcinoma in situ (n=2), stage I breast cancer (n=1), stage I non small cell lung cancer (n=1), colon cancer (n=1) and cholangiocarcinoma (n=1). One further patient had a synchronous papillary bladder cancer at presentation.

Thirty woman were treated in a curative intent for primary cancer of vagina (n=15), cervix (n=9), vulva (n=2) or Bartholin's gland (n=4). Two-thirds of vaginal tumorswere stage II and the majority of malignancies arising in the vulva or in the Bartholin gland was stage III. Among patients affected by a cervical primary cancer, there were 1 stage IIB, 2 stage IIIA, 3 stage IIIB and 3 stage IVA.

Eight other patients who presented with a local recurrence of gynaecological malignancy of the endometrium (n=3), cervix (n=2), vagina (n=1) or vulva (n=2) underwent HDR-ISBT. Two of these patients were treated with brachytherapy with palliative intent. Median time between the last treatment received and the diagnosis of the current recurrence was 11.8 months (IQR: 5.1-39.5 months).

The majority of patients presented either with a squamous cell carcinoma (n=23) or had adenocarcinoma (n=8). The other tumor histologies were adenosquamous carcinoma (n=1), seropapillary adenocarcinoma (n=1), non-keratinizing large cell carcinoma (n=1), basocellular carcinoma (n=1), adenoid cystic carcinoma (n=1), endometrial stromal sarcoma (n=1) and small cell carcinoma (n=1).

Table 1. Patient and tumor characteristics

Characteristics	Overall	Primary Tumor			Recurrence
		Uterine cervix	Vagina	Vulva*	
	n (%)	(n=9)	(n=15)	(n=6)	(n=8)
Age (years)					
Median	56.5	50.0	62.0	53.5	71.0
Range	34-82	44-60	34-82	49-59	49-79
Parity					
0	5 (13)	2	0	2	1
≥1	33 (87)	7	15	4	7
Menauposal status					
Pre-menopausal	7 (18)	4	2	1	0
Post-menopausal	27 (72)	4	11	5	7
Unknown	4 (10)	1	2	0	1
Smoking status					
Current	8 (21)	3	4	1	0
Former	6 (16)	4	0	2	0
Never	23 (60)	2	11	3	7
Unknown	1 (3)	0	0	0	1
FIGO stage					
I	2 (7)	0	2	0	NA
II	12 (40)	1	10	1	NA
III	13 (43)	5	3	5	NA
IV	3 (10)	3	0	0	NA
Histology					
SCC	23 (61)	8	11	2	2
ADK	8 (21)	1	2	1	4
Others	7 (18)	0	2	3	2
Tumor Grade					
G1	10 (26)	2	4	3	1
G2	11 (29)	3	5	0	3
G3	11 (29)	0	6	1	4
Unknown	6 (16)	4	0	2	0
≤ 4 cm	19 (50)	1	7	4	7
> 4 cm	19 (50)	8	8	2	1
LN involvement					
Pelvic	9 (30)	5	4	0	NA
Para-aortic	3 (10)	3	0	0	NA
Inguinal	1 (3)	0	1	0	NA
None	18 (60)	3	9	6	NA
Unknown	2 (7)	1	1	0	NA

Vulva* = vulvar and Bartholin's gland cancer; SCC = squamous cell carcinoma; ADK = adenocarcinoma; LN involvement = lymph node involvement; NA = not applicable/ not available.

Overall treatment characteristics

Dose parameters for EBRT were collected. All patients received pelvic EBRT of 40 to 50.4 Gy given in 1.8-2 Gy per fraction without a midline block. Among the 33 patients receiving the combined radiation therapy, whole pelvis irradiation technique was recorded in 82% of cases. Fifteen patients were treated with parallel opposed fields (AP/PA) and eight with a four field box technique. EBRT was delivered with concurrent chemotherapy in 61 % of cases. All patients affected by a cervical malignancy received concurrent weekly cisplatin at a dose of 40 mg/m^2.

Median overall treatment time for the combined radiation treatment, consisting of EBRT plus HDR-ISBT, was 59 days (IQR: 52-76 days). Median time between the end of EBRT and the beginning of HDR-ISBT was 20 days (IQR: 12-37 days).

DVH parameters

The median volume of CTV was 84.9 cc (IQR: 62.5-106.4 cc). The median EQD$_2$ D90 and D100 were 89.2 Gy$_{10}$ (IQR: 85.2-92.3 Gy$_{10}$) and 68.5 Gy$_{10}$ (IQR: 65.5-71.9 Gy$_{10}$) respectively. The median V100 was 97.5% (IQR: 96.4-98.4%). The median V150 and V200 were 32.5 cc (IQR: 24.4-40.9 cc) and 13.0 cc (IQR: 8.5-14.9 cc). The median HI was 0.61 (IQR: 0.54-0.67).

Table 2 shows the dose-volume values for OARs. The median contoured rectal, bladder and urethral volume were respectively 67.6 cc (IQR: 48.4-90.5 cc), 58.6 cc (IQR: 35.7-69.8 cc) and 0.9 cc (IQR: 0.7-1.2 cc). The median D$_{2cc}$ for rectum and bladder were 80.1 Gy$_3$ (IQR: 71.8-85.7 Gy$_3$) and 76.9 Gy$_3$ (IQR: 71.4-81.5 Gy$_3$). The median D$_{0.1cc}$ and D10 for urethra were 79.7 Gy$_3$ (IQR: 68.6-97.0 Gy$_3$) and 79.5 Gy$_3$ (IQR: 69.0-95.4 Gy$_3$).

Table 2. Dose-volume parameters of the OARs (EQD$_2$, Gy$_{\alpha/\beta=3}$)

Organ at risk	Median	Lower Quartile	Upper Quartile
Rectum			
D$_{0.1cc}$	94.9	84.0	105.8
D$_{1cc}$	84.3	74.9	90.5
D$_{2cc}$	80.1	71.8	85.7
Bladder			
D$_{0.1cc}$	92.4	85.7	107.2
D$_{1cc}$	81.2	74.6	87.5
D$_{2cc}$	76.9	71.4	81.5
Urethra			
D$_{0.1cc}$	79.7	68.6	97.0
D10	79.5	69.0	95.4

D$_{0.1cc}$, D$_{1cc}$, D$_{2cc}$ = minimum dose for the most irradiated 0.1, 1, 2 cc, respectively; D10 = the dose to 10% volume of the contoured urethra.

Response to Treatment and Tumor Control

Median follow-up was 20.6 months (IQR: 8.9-37.9 months) for all patients, and respectively 28.0 and 8.7 months for those with primary and recurrent tumors.

Out of the 36 patients for whom response to treatment was reported, 92% had a favourable response. Rate of complete response (CR), partial response (PR) and stable disease (SD) after HDR-ISBT were respectively 85.71%, 10.71% and 3.57% for primary tumors compared to 75%, 0 and 25% for recurrent cancers (p=0.226). Among patients who achieved a CR, six had a subsequent local recurrence (2 primary cancers; 4 recurrent diseases). Among patients with a PR or SD, two suffered from a local progression (2 primary cancers). Median time between the end of the HDR-ISBT and the occurrence of a local failure was 7.9 months (IQR: 5.6-14.2 months). Local control for primary and recurrent malignancies, shown in Figure 3, was respectively 86.6% versus 37.5% at 2 years and 81.3% versus 37.5% at 5 years (p=0.0066). Throughout follow-up, 7 women with a primary malignancy develop a regional or distal recurrence, including 3 patients who had only a partial response assessed after brachytherapy, 1 patient diagnosed with a vaginal grade 3 small cell carcinoma and 1 patient with a past stage IIIC colon cancer. In parallel, four patients treated with HDR-ISBT for a recurrent tumorexperienced a distant failure.

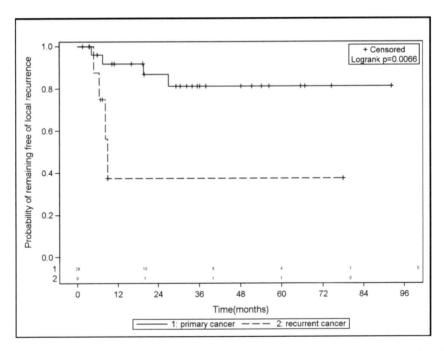

Figure 3. Clinical local control rates for primary and recurrent gynaecologic malignancies after high-dose-rate interstitial brachytherapy

Table 3. Univariate predictors of complete response to treatment

Variable	OR	95% CI	p-value
Age (<60 vs ≥60 years)	0.35	0.007-3.80	0.66
Current smoking (yes vs no)	2.37	0.29-∞	0.46
Tumor size (≤4 vs >4 cm)	0.45	0.04-3.69	0.66
Volume of CTV (≤100 vs >100 cc)	1.16	0.09-9.95	1.00
Hemoglobin levels (<120 vs ≥120 g/L)	0.77	0.09-6.73	1.00
Primary vs Recurrent malignancy	1.96	0.15-18.04	0.81
Timing of EBRT (past vs prior to HDR-ISBT)	0.24	0.02-3.63	0.37
Overall treatment time (≤ 8 vs >8 weeks)	1.38	0.09-22.15	1.00
Time between EBRT and HDR-ISBT (≤15 vs >15 days)	2.18	0.15-131.03	0.94
Chemotherapy concomitant to EBRT (yes vs no)	1.67	0.11-26.47	1.00
D90 (<87 vs ≥87 Gy_{10})	1.06	0.12-13.83	1.00
D100 (<66 vs ≥66 Gy_{10})	1.45	0.17-18.76	1.00
In primary gynecologic malignancies:			
Stage (I-II vs III-IV)	0.85	0.05-13.58	1.00
Grade (I-II vs III)	1.08	0.02-24.82	1.00
Histology (SCC vs ADK)	1.73	0.03-33.34	1.00
Initial site (others vs cervix)	2.35	0.14-38.57	0.77
Initial site (vagina vs others)	0.85	0.05-13.58	1.00

OR= exact odds ratio; EBRT = external beam radiation therapy; HDR-ISBT = high-dose-rate interstitial brachytherapy; SCC = squamous cell carcinoma; ADK = adenocarcinoma.

Table 4. Univariate predictors of the absence of local recurrences

Variable	OR	95% CI	p-value
Age (<60 vs ≥60 years)	1.08	0.14-7.00	1.00
Current smoking (yes vs no)	1.97	0.18-104.9	0.97
Tumor size (≤4 vs >4 cm)	0.53	0.07-3.35	0.69
Volume of CTV (≤100 vs >100 cc)	0.15	0-1.15	0.07
Hemoglobin levels (<120 vs ≥120 g/L)	0.66	0.10-4.31	0.88
Primary vs Recurrent malignancy	5.62	0.74-47.16	0.11
Timing of EBRT (past vs prior to HDR-ISBT)	0.14	0.009-1.53	0.12
Overall treatment time (≤ 8 vs >8 weeks)	0.48	0.008-7.02	0.96
Time between EBRT and HDR-ISBT (≤15 vs >15 days)	0.22	0.004-3.27	0.42
Chemotherapy concomitant to EBRT (yes vs no)	2.73	0.26-38.46	0.56
D90 (<87 vs ≥87 Gy_{10})	1.39	0.18-17.47	1.00
D100 (<66 vs ≥66 Gy_{10})	1.93	0.25-23.91	0.78
In primary gynecologic malignancies:			
Stage (I-II vs III-IV)	0.85	0.05-13.57	1.00
Grade (I-II vs III)	5.11	0.22-353.3	0.45
Histology (SCC vs ADK)	14.31	0.54-∞	0.13
Initial site (others vs cervix)	0.82	0.01-12.39	1.00
Initial site (vagina vs others)	0.29	0.005-4.29	0.59

OR= exact odds ratio; EBRT = external beam radiation therapy; HDR-ISBT = high-dose-rate interstitial brachytherapy; SCC = squamous cell carcinoma; ADK = adenocarcinoma.

Univariate analyses were done to explore the association between possible predictive factors and complete response to treatment (Table 3) or the absence of local recurrence (Table 4). Univariate analysis shown in Tables 3 and 4 didn't reveal any significant association. A non-significant trend is observed for the larger CTV where a contoured volume exceeding 100cc leads to a better local tumor control.

Survival

Disease-free survival (DFS) was significantly longer in the primary cancer group than in the recurrent cancer group (p=0.003). At 2 years, the rate of DFS was 68.6% (95% CI = 46.3 to 83.1%) in the primary cancer group and 18.8% (95% CI = 1.1 to 53.5%) in the recurrent cancer group, as shown in Figure 4. Figure 5 shows the Kaplan-Meier curves for overall survival (OS). The 5 year-OS was 78.9% (95% CI = 55.4 to 90.9%) for primary tumors compared to 14.3% (95% CI = 0.7 to 46.5%) for recurrences. The log-rank test revealed a statistically significant difference between the OS rates over time (p<0.001). Median survival time had not been reached for primary malignancies but it was 8.8 months for recurrent gynaecologic cancers. Nine women died of their gynaecologic malignancy, one died of a metastastic disease either secondary to her current vaginal carcinoma or a past colon cancer and another patient died of an acute upper gastrointestinal bleeding secondary to a gastric vascular malformation. The Kaplan-Meier estimates of the 2 and 5-year disease-specific survival rates for the primary cancer group (n=30) were respectively 91.3% (95% CI = 69.5 to 97.8%) and 84.8% (95% CI = 58.9 to 95.0%).

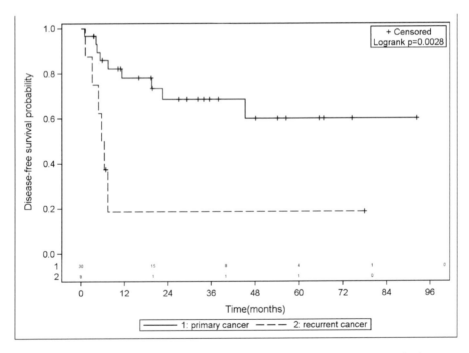

Figure 4. Disease-free survival curve of 38 patients with primary or recurrent gynaecologic cancer.

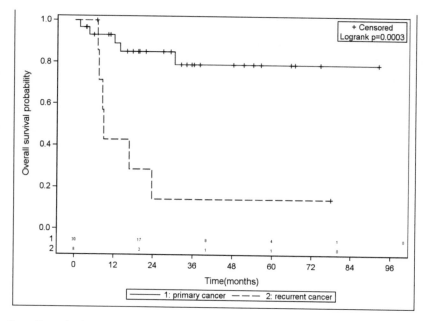

Figure 5. Overall survival curve of 38 patients with primary or recurrent gynaecologic cancer.

Adverse Effects

No complication occurred at implantation or extraction. Seventy-four percent of patients experienced grade 1 or grade 2 acute toxicity. Grade 2 rectal mucositis, diarrhea, urethral burning and vaginal mucositis were noted in 2, 1, 5 and 9 patients, respectively. Six patients developed grade 3 vaginal mucositis and 3 had vaginal necrosis. Two of these last 9 women affected by a vaginal toxicity had also a grade 3 acute urethral burning. Fortunately, vaginal acute necrosis resolved completely in two of three women. Only one of them was still affected by necrosis as a late effect.

Table 5 lists the late toxicities seen in the study population. Grade 3-4 late toxicities were observed in 12 patients. No grade 5 toxicity occurred. A total of 9 patients experienced vaginal necrosis: 4 grade 2 necrosis managed with local wound care and 5 grade 3 necrosis treated with hyperbaric oxygen. The vaginal necrosis slowly resolved in 7 of the 9 patients. The two patients who remain with vaginal necrosis at last follow-up were the one previously discussed having acute necrosis and a woman treated in 2001 who experienced several serious complications after 50.4 Gy by EBRT and 18 Gy in 3 fractions by HDR-ISBT. This last woman suffered from a grade 3 cystitis, had a transient grade 3 diarrhea due to radiation induced ileitis and she subsequently required the resection of the distal ileum for intestinal obstruction. Paradoxically, she was the patient who received the lowest HDR-ISBT doses in the whole group. Her DVH parameters were not recorded unfortunately for our dose-volume study. At the cost of severe complications, this patient is still alive free of disease. Another patient, for whom the dosimetric data were unavailable, experienced urethral stenosis. Among the 11 patients who were detected with needle perforation of the bladder at the time of the post-implant cystoscopy or CT-scan, none developed acute or late cystitis and only 1 experienced late urethral burning. One more patient, without bladder puncture, had grade 2 late urethral burning.

Table 6 summaries the dose-volume parameters of patients who developed a grade 2 to 4 late gastrointestinal (GI) morbidity and reports the evolution of these toxicities, considering toxicities registered at the last follow-up. Seven of these 9 patients received chemotherapy concomitant to EBRT. Their median rectal D_{2cc} was 81.6 Gy_3, which was similar to 80.1 Gy_3, the median D_{2cc} of the study population. However, their median for $D_{0.1cc}$, 103.7 Gy_3, was higher than the one of the whole group, 94.9 Gy_3. This substantial difference in $D_{0.1cc}$ values could suggest a dose-effect relationship. Although the incidence of grade 2-4 late GI toxicity was relatively high, morbidity was transient and only one woman was still suffering from a grade 2 GI toxicity at last follow-up.

Table 5. Worst grade late toxicities

Toxicity	Grade (No. of patients)			
	1	2	3	4
Gastrointestinal				
Rectal ulcer	0	4	1	0
Bleeding	5	4	1	0
Diarrhea	6	2	1	0
Incontinence	0	1	0	0
Small bowel obstruction	0	0	0	1
Urinary				
Cystitis	0	0	1	0
Urethral burning	0	2	0	0
Urethral stenosis	0	0	1	0
Incontinence	5	1	0	0
Others				
Vaginal mucositis	0	2	1	9
Fistula	0	0	0	1

Table 6. DVH parameters of patients affected by a grade 2-4 late GI toxicity

Pt	Dosimetry		Late GI toxicity	
	$RD_{0.1cc}$ (Gy$_3$)	RD_{2cc} (Gy$_3$)	Worst grade	Last visit
1	NA	NA	Grade 4 small bowel obstruction, grade 3 diarrhea	None
2	NA	NA	Grade 2 fecal incontinence	None
3	75.6	69.3	Grade 2 bleeding	Grade 2 bleeding
4	105.8	80.3	Grade 2 rectal ulcer	None
5	106.6	84.1	Grade 2 rectal ulcer	Grade 1 diarrhea
6	133.3	91.8	Grade 2 bleeding	Grade 1 bleeding
7	92.9	76.2	Grade 3 rectal ulcer, grade 2 bleeding	Grade 1 bleeding
8	97.6	81.6	Grade 4 recto-vaginal fistula, grade 2 rectal ulcer, grade 2 bleeding, grade 2 diarrhea	Grade 1 diarrhea
9	103.7	83.3	Grade 3 bleeding, grade 2 rectal ulcer, grade 2 diarrhea	Grade 1 bleeding, grade 1 diarrhea

GI = gastrointestinal; Pt = patient; $RD_{0.1cc}$, RD_{2cc} = minimum dose for the most irradiated 0.1 and 2 cc of the rectum, respectively; NA = not available.

In summary, the vast majority of patients had improvement or resolution of their late toxicities. Only two patients were suffering from grade 3-4 toxicity (vaginal necrosis) at the last follow-up visit.

On univariate analysis, there was no statistically significant relationship between the clinical variables and the occurrence of grade 3-4 acute or late toxicity.

Discussion

Therapeutic management of gynaecologic malignancies is challenging and HDR-ISBT seems to be a reasonable modality to achieve a good local control and survival when intracavitary brachytherapy cannot adequately cover the target volume or reach the optimal dose distribution. Indications for gynaecologic ISBT according to the ABS [5-6, 20] are:

1. A narrow or distorted vagina,
2. The incapacity to insert a tandem in the endocervical canal for cervix cancer,
3. A bulky primary disease,
4. An extensive parametrial or vaginal involvement,
5. A tumorthickness >5 mm after the completion of EBRT,
6. A persistent disease after EBRT and intracavitary implant,
7. A gynaecologic cancer recurrence after hysterectomy, and
8. Simply for previously irradiated patients.

As demonstrated in this chapter, a favourable response can be achieve in up to 96% and 75% of patients affected by primary and recurrent gynaecologic malignancies, respectively. Long-term local control can be expected in more than 80% of cases for primary tumors using inverse planning for CT-based HDR-ISBT. The delivery of high doses of radiation has many potential advantages but patient should be advised that severe toxicities may occur. These toxicities are transient in most patients but may persist long term in rare cases. Valid dose volume constraints must be applied for safety.

Use of 3D Planning

MRI is known to be superior to other imaging modalities through its multiplanar capacity and its high soft tissue resolution for delineating gynaecologic tumors, identifying parametrial or vaginal tumor extension and for imaging the normal pelvic organs [21-22]. Figure 6 shows MRI images of a gynaecologic interstitial implant performed at our institution. Although MRI has allowed great advances in gynaecologic cancer imaging, its use for 3D gynaecologic brachytherapy treatment planning remains marginal in North America. CT is the preferred modality. Indeed, a recent survey among the ABS members reports that only 2% of the respondents use MRI images to assist for treatment planning while 55% and 43 % reported using CT and plain films as their imaging modality for target dose specification, respectively [3]. A number of constraints explain the sparse use of MRI guidance, including the high cost and limited availability of MRI, the need of nonmagnetic applicators and the increase amount of time required by physicians.

CT-based brachytherapy represents the actual pattern of practice in North America but literature is rare considering CT-based HDR-ISBT. According to our review of the published English-language literature, less than fifteen studies report the use of HDR-ISBT and even fewer presented clinical outcomes exclusive to external beam radiation combined with HDR-ISBT [23-35]. Briefly, all these studies have a limited number of patients and various doses per fraction, total doses, templates, dose specification and optimization methods were employed. Of these, the majority used 2D planning. Few studies concern CT-based HDR-ISBT and only 2 are related to MRI assistance for implantation or planning. Viswanathan et al. [28] describe the use of real-time MRI guidance during the implant procedure and CT imaging regarding treatment planning and dose specification. Yoshida et al. [32] recently published on CT-based planning with MRI assistance to contour the HR-CTV and OARs. Some other studies on combined intracavitary and interstitial brachytherapy are available but are not the focus of the current chapter. Nevertheless, we acknowledge the work of Kim et al. [36] for presenting the first clinical outcomes using IPSA for cervical cancer MRI-guided intracavitary brachytherapy with or without interstitial needles.

The anatomy-based IPSA algorithm was used in this chapter in order to optimize the dose distribution. The inverse treatment planning system automatically activates selective dwell positions and find the optimal dwell time combination to best fulfill the dosimetric objectives, taking into account the clinical target and all organs at risk [16].

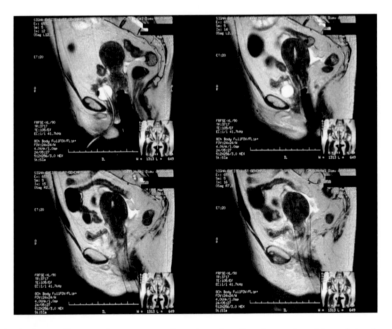

Figure 6. Sagittal views of magnetic resonance imaging showing the perineal template, the vaginal guide, interstitial needles and a Foley catheter.

In this chapter, we are one of the first to report clinical outcomes and dose-volume parameters using IPSA regarding CT-based HDR-ISBT for gynaecologic malignancies, one of the first to investigate DVH parameters of OARs recommended by the Gyn GEC-ESTRO and recorded with the total doses in EQD$_2$ for CT-based gynaecologic HDR-ISBT and one of the first to present urethral dose-volume parameters values for gynaecologic HDR-ISBT.

Clinical Outcomes

Table 7 summaries clinical outcomes reported in the literature regarding gynaecologic HDR-ISBT. All those patients also received pelvic EBRT or prior irradiation. As mentioned, data are heterogeneous and sparse. In short, a complete response rate can be achieved in 75 to 90 % of patients with a primary gynaecologic cancer and in 22.7 to 80% in patients with a recurrent gynaecologic cancer. We obtained favorable or at least equivalent results compared to those previously published, with CR rates of 85.7% and 75% for primary and recurrent malignancies. Five-year local control rate between 64 to 94% can be reached for primary tumors and we obtained 81.3%. However, as demonstrated in this chapter and by Itami et al. [24], less than 50% of patients affected by a recurrence will remain free of local recurrence at 2 years.

Table 7. Comparison of clinical outcomes after
HDR-ISBT between studies

Study	No. of patients	Primary tumor site or R	HDR-ISBT Dose per fraction (Gy)	No. of fractions	CR rate (%)	5-year LC (%)
Demanes et al.	62	Cervix	5.5-6	4-6	NA	94
Itami et al.	17	Gyn and R	4-6	NA	NA	75 and 47*
Susworo et al.	9	Cervix and R	2-10	2-8	75 and 80	NA
Sitathanee et al.	10	Cervix and Vagina	5-7.5	1-6	90	NA
Beriwal et al.	16	Cervix and Vagina	3.75	5	81	75
Nandwani et al.	85	Gyn	4	4-6	NA	64.7
Badakd et al.	22	R	4-6	2-9	22.7	NA
Isohashi et al.	25	Cervix	6	5	NA	73 (stage III)
Current results	38	Gyn and R	4-6	3-7	85.7 and 75	81.3 and 37.5

HDR-ISBT = high-dose-rate interstitial brachtherapy; R = recurrent gynaecologic cancer; CR = complete response; LC = local control; NA = non available; Gyn = multiple gynaecologic tumor sites; * = 2-year local control.

The great heterogeneity of the published results for HDR-ISBT and for LDR-ISBT makes it also difficult to compare the two techniques. Local control rates described in the literature for LDR-ISBT range from 25% to 100%, and are especially between 50-80% [37-44].

In the series of Kim et al. [36], the estimated probability of 2-year local control was 96% in cervical cancer patients treated with HDR brachytherapy using IPSA for MRI-based planning. They used tandem and ovoids or tandem and cylinder with or without additional interstitial needles. In comparison, we achieve 86.6% of local control at 2 years in patients affected by a primary tumor, which we believe is excellent considering that all these patients were unsuitable for intracavitary brachytherapy.

A dose-response correlation was identified recently by Dimopoulos et al. [45] between local control rates and dose-volume parameters of the HR-CTV in MRI-guided intracavitary brachytherapy. Local control was defined in their study as the absence of tumorwithin the true pelvis. They reported on 141 patients with cervical cancer. Mean total doses in EQD_2 for D90 and D100 were significantly higher in patients without local recurrences than in patients affected by a local recurrence (87 vs 75 Gy_{10} and 66 vs 60 Gy_{10}; p<0.05). These values were used as cut-off limits for the respective DVH parameters. They demonstrated that 3-year local control could be achieved in >95% of patients if a D90 ≥87 Gy_{10} for HR-CTV could be reached. Likewise, a D100 ≥66 Gy_{10} for the HR-CTV resulted in a local control rate exceeding 87%, irrespective of tumor size. Furthermore, they established that the dose at which a local control rate of 90% could be expected was 86 Gy_{10} for the D100 and 67 Gy_{10} for the D90 HR-CTV [46].

On univariate analysis, we didn't observe for CT-based HDR-ISBT any of these correlations between D90 ≥87 Gy_{10} or a D100 ≥66 Gy_{10} for the CTV and either a complete response noted after brachytherapy or long-term local control probability. Our median D90 and D100 for CTV were 89.2 Gy_{10} and 68.5 Gy_{10}, respectively. Similarly, we didn't observe any statistically significant predictive factor on univariate analysis which could be explained mostly by our small sample size and consequently the lack of power.

Yoshida et al. [32] reported their experience with MRI assistance for 3D-based HDR-ISBT in 18 patients diagnosed with uterine cervical malignancy. Their median D90 and D100 for HR-CTV were 80.6 Gy_{10} and 62.4 Gy_{10} (EQD_2). Local recurrence occurred in 3 patients (17%) after a median follow-up of 18 months. For the 3 patients, the median D90 and D100 HR-CTV were 81.9 Gy_{10} and 53.9 Gy_{10} and no significant statistical difference was detected.

In summary, 3D image-based HDR-ISBT is indicated when intracavitary might not sufficiently encompass the gynaecologic tumor. Even in these patients with unfavourable disease, good local control can be expected, namely higher than 80%. For now, no dose-response correlation was demonstrated for HDR-ISBT, but it would be reasonable to use cut-off values reported by Dimopoulos et al. [45-46] for HDR intracavitary brachytherapy.

Adverse Effects

Late toxicities are a major concern for patients who underwent gynaecologic interstitial brachytherapy because the reported incidence of adverse effects was traditionally higher than with intracavitary brachytherapy. Twelve patients experienced a grade 3-4 late morbidity in this chapter but toxicity was transient, regressing or resolving in 83% of them. Therefore, only two patients have suffered from a chronic severe late effect. This proportion of patients experiencing a transient grade 3-4 late toxicity may seem relatively high compared to the rates reported so far, but comparisons should be made with caution due to the heterogeneity of published data. Reported severe complication rates after gynaecologic HDR-ISBT range from 6.5% to 23.5% [23-32], depending on the way the event is defined, the scoring system used to grade toxicity, the cumulative dose received, EBRT and brachytherapy techniques, the localization of the tumor and the follow-up of the population.

Demanes et al. [23] noted 6.5% of chronic grade 3-4 morbidity in their study population. Before HDR-ISBT, patients received 25-36 Gy to the pelvis by EBRT using a four field technique and additional EBRT was delivered between brachytherapy applications to the pelvic sidewalls, with a midline block and AP/PA fields. Treatment planning for brachytherapy was 2D. Morbidity consisted of one vesicovaginal fistula, one vaginal necrosis leading to a fatal hemorrhage and two cases of small bowel obstruction.

In their series, Itami et al. [24] identified 4 grade 4 late complications (23.5%) according to the SOMA grading system. Mean dose of pelvic EBRT given was 35.4 Gy and mean dose of HDR-ISBT was 26.2 Gy. In comparison, we delivered between 40-50.4 Gy to the pelvis with EBRT and a median dose of 30Gy by HDR-ISBT. Among their 17 patients, those with a tumor volume exceeding 100 cm^3 had a significantly higher incidence of grade 2-4 toxicities, with 78% of toxicity versus 0 for cancer ≤ 100 cm^3.

Beriwal et al. [27] reported their complications using the Radiation Therapy Oncology Group (RTOG) scales. Sixteen patients with vaginal or cervical primary malignancies were treated with EBRT and HDR-ISBT for 5 fractions of 3.75Gy. They received thus a cumulative biologically effective dose (BED) of 78.9 Gy_{10} to the tumor, corresponding to 65.8 Gy_{10} in EQD_2. Five of them (31%) experienced grade ≥ 2 late morbidity.

In the series of Isohashi et al. [31], 25 patients were treated with CT-based HDR-ISBT to a median BED of 84 Gy_{10} to the target volume, corresponding to 70 Gy_{10} in EQD_2. Twelve percent (12%) of the patients developed grade 2 or higher late toxicity. The median V150 and V200 were 32 cc (range: 8-75 cc) and 7.5 cc (range: 3-11 cc) while our results showed values of 32.5 cc (range: 14-80 cc) and 13 cc (range: 5.5-36.8 cc), respectively.

Badakh et al. [30] observed 4 grade 4 complications out of 22 patients (18%) treated with HDR-ISBT, graded with the LENT SOMA scales.

Shah et al. [35] recently reported that 5.6% and 8.3% of their population respectively had genitourinary and GI grade 3-4 late morbidity after LDR- or HDR-ISBT, consisting of 4 fractions of 5-6 Gy, using CT planning. They also demonstrated the absence of relationship between needle puncture of bladder or bowel and the occurrence of acute or late toxicity. We present in this chapter results confirming this finding. None of the patients in which bladder perforation occurred during implantation developed acute or late cystitis or hematuria.

The rate of adverse effects observed for HDR-ISBT seems also quite similar to those reported in the literature for LDR interstitial brachytherapy. The general incidence of severe complications described for LDR-ISBT range from to 10 to 21% [37-44]. In their series, Aristizabal et al. [13] and Ampuero et al. [47] even identified increased rate of severe toxicity of 33% and 42%, respectively.

The high incidence of severe late toxicities in this chapter is mainly related to the occurrence of vaginal necrosis that we considered as a grade 4 vaginal mucositis regardless of the area affected. Interestingly, the nine patients who developed necrosis were treated before 2006 and we believe these complications may be relative to the learning curve to perform the implant and in determination of optimization parameters. Moreover, it may be relative to the evolving knowledge and the scientific evidence for dose-volume constraints, used for inverse planning calculations. One patient developed unexpectedly large number of severe toxicities despite small doses delivered with brachytherapy, including vaginal necrosis, late GI and urinary morbidities. This patient could have had a particularly higher radiosensibility than the general population.

Over time, necrosis completely resolved in 7 of the 9 women, with local wound care or with hyperbaric oxygen. Likewise, severe GI late morbidities were transient. As reported by Faria et al. [48], adverse effects that slowly resolved with time or with appropriate treatment are fairly less significant than toxicities that last and become chronic. This distinction must be considered when evaluating toxicities. Toxicity severity may vary over time and adequate assessment of adverse effects relies on multiple visits and a minimum follow-up. Furthermore, grading may differ depending on the subjectivity of the physician.

Dose-Volume Parameters for the Oars

Rectum and bladder

In this chapter, we performed a dosimetric evaluation using the 3D-based DVH parameters proposed by the Gyn GEC-ESTRO for the rectum and bladder. $D_{0.1cc}$, D_{1cc} and D_{2cc} are recommended for reporting, and optionally also D_{5cc} and D_{10cc}, derived from MRI-based treatment planning in cervix cancer intracavitary brachytherapy[17]. No such guidelines exist for interstitial brachytherapy, neither for using CT. However, Viswanathan et al. [49] demonstrated that there were no significant difference in DVH parameters values using the Gyn GEC-ESTRO recommendations between CT and MRI contours for intracavitary brachytherapy with or without interstitial needles. In assessing DVH parameters for the OARs, we chose to record $D_{0.1cc}$, D_{1cc} and D_{2cc}, because it has been shown that the DVHs computed were almost identicals for external organ contours and organ wall contouring when volumes smaller than 5 cc are considered. When volumes $\geq$ 5 cc are evaluated, difference in bladder and rectal filling invalidated this correspondence [17, 50].

Our DVH parameters values of rectum and bladder are compared with the results of others studies [32, 51-53] in Table 8 considering the total doses received to 2 cc. Our results for the bladder are similar to previous reports and even favourable compared to the median D_{2cc} value of the multicenter intercomparison study by Lang et al., a validation study that showed that different treatment concepts could be compared between institutions, using the Gyn GEC-ESTRO guidelines for MRI[51]. The results for the bladder D_{2cc} were also similar to those of the University of California, San Francisco published by Kubicky et al. [54], that performed IPSA from MRI for cervix cancer intracavitary brachytherapy. They obtained in 15 patients a mean $D_{0.1cc}$, D_{1cc} and D_{2cc} of 91, 78 and 74 Gy_3 for bladder and of 79, 70 and 67 Gy_3 for rectum, respectively. The somewhat higher values of our rectal D_{2cc} can be explained by the proximity of the rectum to our target volume since we included vaginal malignancies and gynaecologic recurrence while others studies only looked at primary uterine cervical cancer. Furthermore, we conducted a retrospective study on patients treated since 2001 and obviously, dose-volume constraints for OARs were not systematically set to fulfill the 2006 Gyn GEC-ESTRO recommendations[17].

Even if 3D-based DVH parameters established by the Gyn GEC-ESTRO for OARs seem to be appropriate to compare treatment plans, a main interrogation is whether these DVH values have a clinical correlation with late toxicities. We have pointed out in this chapter a noticeable difference in rectal $D_{0.1cc}$ values between patients who experienced a transient grade 2-4 GI late toxicity and the median of the whole study population. However, this difference was not found for rectal D_{2cc}. Up to now, few data support a dose-effect correlation between dose-volume parameters and clinical late bladder and rectum toxicities, but clear association was demonstrated for endoscopic rectal mucosal changes and rectal morbidity. Koom et al. [52] noted a significant association between $D_{0.1cc}$, D_{1cc}, D_{2cc} and the endoscopic scoring of rectal mucosal changes. Formation of telangiectatic vessels was the most important parameter evaluated in that study because telangiectasia has been found to be related to late fibrosis and necrosis. Georg et al. [55] on their side identified significant higher dose values for $D_{0.1cc}$, D_{1cc} and D_{2cc} in patients with clinical symptoms and endoscopic changes compared to asymptomatic patients. They also estimated the dose at which clinical symptoms would be expected in 50% of the patient treated with combined EBRT and intracavitary brachytherapy (ED50) and it was $76Gy_3$ for the rectal D_{2cc}. This finding however was not corroborated by our results with HDR-ISBT.

Further prospective studies are necessary to assess the dose-effect relationships for intracavitary and for interstitial brachytherapy. For now, the recommendations for rectal D_{2cc} constraint are around 75 Gy_3 in cervix cancer intracavitary brachytherapy. It relies mainly on the documented correlation observed between D_{2cc} and the dose at the ICRU rectal reference point (D_{ICRU}) and on the previously established association between D_{ICRU} and the risk of rectal late complications. On the contrary, no such relationships exist for the bladder. Dose constraints of 80 to 95 Gy_3 were used for the bladder D_{2cc} but no bladder dose-volume constraint is currently defined [17, 55-58].

**Table 8. Comparison of dose parameters values
for OARs between studies (EQD$_2$, Gy$_{\alpha/\beta=3}$)**

	Interstitial Brachytherapy		Intracavitary Brachytherapy		
	Our results	Yoshida et al.	Lang et al.	Koom et al.	Beriwal et al.
	(38 pts)	(18 pts)	(3 pts)	(71 pts)	(10 pts)
OAR	Median (range)	Median (range)	Median (range)	Mean (± SD)	Mean (range)
Rectum					
D_{2cc}	80.1 (57.8-91.8)	65.9 (48.9-76)	62 (53-64)	67 (± 9)	56.6 (51.5-64.6)
Bladder					
D_{2cc}	76.9 (58.9-101.5)	62 (51.4-89)	81 (70-85)	84 (± 15)	75.0 (61.8-81.6)
Imaging modality	CT	MRI assistance	MRI	CT	MRI and CT

OAR = organ at risk; pts = patients; SD = standard deviation; D_{2cc} = the minimum dose for the most irradiated 2 cc of the respective organ; CT = computed tomography; MRI = magnetic resonance imaging.

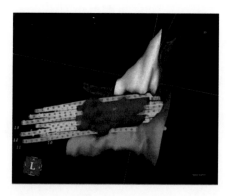

Figure 7. Three-dimensional computed image reconstruction of the catheters, target volume and organs at risk contours in a gynaecologic implant. Catheters = sky blue or green; Target volume = blue; Bladder = white; Rectum = pink; Urethra and small bowel = in blue, on each side of the bladder.

Urethra

This chapter is the first to report DVH values of the urethra in gynaecologic HDR-ISBT. We have chosen to record $D_{0.1cc}$ and D10 for assessment of DVH parameters because previous recommendations have supported their use for prostate cancer brachytherapy. The GEC-ESTRO and the European Association of Urology (EAU) proposed in 2005 to use $D_{0.1cc}$ or D1 for reporting dose to urethra in prostate HDR-ISBT [59]. In 2007, the GEC-ESTRO recommended a urethral D10 inferior to 150% of the prescription dose as the primary parameter to consider for the urethra in permanent seed prostate brachytherapy. Secondary parameters suggested were urethral $D_{0.1cc}$, D5 and D30 [60]. We delineated the urethra contour using the visible urethral catheter on all CT slices where clinical target volume was identified. Urethra and others OARs contouring is shown in Figure 7. Interestingly, the two patients who had grade 2 late urethral burning had higher dose-volume values for urethra than the median value of the study population, with values of 97.0 Gy_3 and 99.5 Gy_3 compared to 79.7 Gy_3 for urethral $D_{0.1cc}$ and with values of 94.0 Gy_3 and 100.5 Gy_3 compared to 79.5 Gy_3 for the D10. Our results show similarity between the median $D_{0.1cc}$ (79.7 Gy_3) and D10 (79.5 Gy_3). This finding correlates with the mean difference of 1% identified by Kirisits et al. [61] between the urethral $D_{0.1cc}$ and D10 for patients treated with prostate HDR boost. Comparison with the published literature concerning doses is for now limited because urethral $D_{0.1cc}$ and D10 values were rarely recorded in EQD_2 cumulative dose, consisting of EBRT and brachytherapy contribution, for prostate cancer. Scientific evidence of a dose-effect correlation between urethral DVH parameters and complications is scarce. However, Akimoto et al. [62] identified a correlation between D10 values and the severity grade of acute genitourinary toxicity after prostate HDR brachytherapy combined with EBRT. Because acute and late urethral morbidity may occur and affect patient quality of life, it is an area of concern and we thus suggest to record and report $D_{0.1cc}$ or D10 in total EQD_2 doses in order to assess and investigate urethral doses for gynaecologic interstitial brachytherapy.

Vagina

While it is well accepted that vagina is a main OAR and that it should be taken into consideration when performing gynaecologic brachytherapy, no dose-volume parameter is currently defined to assess vaginal wall dosimetry. Literature is rare and scientific evidence is lacking on that issue. Nose et al. [63] published on in vivo dosimetry for pelvic HDR-ISBT and they have used in their series the tumor dose to evaluate the vaginal wall dosimetry.

Although clinical outcomes, toxicity and dosimetric evaluation reported in this chapter include limitations inherent to a retrospective design, these results are important due to the limited data published on CT-based HDR-ISBT. This chapter also presents results using IPSA and literature is sparse on that subject. Furthermore, all implants were performed by the same radiation oncologist and all patients were followed up by the same physician, allowing consistency of assessment. Such heterogeneity of the study population is also encountered in other series on HDR-ISBT.

The results described in this chapter and the review of the literature on HDR interstitial brachytherapy have highlighted a delicate balance between doses, local control and adverse effects. Many questions are still unresolved and further studies are required to investigate DVH constraints and clinical outcomes.

Conclusion

In summary, a local control rate higher than 80% can be expected with gynaecologic CT-based HDR-ISBT in patients unsuitable for intracavitary brachytherapy, but transient severe complications may occur and careful attention should be paid to minimize the dose to normal organs and tissues. Until now, no dose-response correlation for local control and no dose-effect relationship were demonstrated for gynaecologic HDR-ISBT, but it is reasonable to rely on the data found for HDR intracavitary brachytherapy. In order to investigate and compare results between institutions, dose-volume parameters for bladder and rectum should be recorded according to the Gyn GEC-ESTRO guidelines, and D10 or $D_{0.1cc}$ should be reported for the urethra in gynaecologic 3D image-based HDR-ISBT. Doses should be normalized in EQD_2.

References

[1]   Tod, MC; Meredith, W. A dosage system for use in the treatment of cancer of the uterine cervix. *Br J Radiol*, 1938, 11, 809-823.

[2]   ICRU. Dose and volume specification for reporting intracavitary therapy in gynecology: Report no 38. Bethesda, MD: *Internationa lCommissionon Radiation Units and Measurements*. 1985.

[3]   Viswanathan, AN; Erickson, BA. Three-dimensional imaging in gynecologic brachytherapy: a survey of the American Brachytherapy Society. *Int J Radiat Oncol Biol Phys.*, 2010, 76, 104-109.

[4]   Haie-Meder, C; Potter, R; Van Limbergen, E; et al. Recommendations from Gynaecological (GYN) GEC-ESTRO Working Group (I): concepts and terms in 3D image based 3D treatment planning in cervix cancer brachytherapy with emphasis on MRI assessment of GTV and CTV. *Radiother Oncol*, 2005, 74, 235-245.

[5]   Nag, S; Erickson, B; Thomadsen, B; Orton, C; Demanes, JD; Petereit, D. The American Brachytherapy Society recommendations for high-dose-rate brachytherapy for carcinoma of the cervix. *Int J Radiat Oncol Biol Phys.*, 2000, 48, 201-211.

[6]   Nag, S; Erickson, B; Parikh, S; Gupta, N; Varia, M; Glasgow, G. The American Brachytherapy Society recommendations for high-dose-rate brachytherapy for carcinoma of the endometrium. *Int J Radiat Oncol Biol Phys.*, 2000, 48, 779-790.

[7]   Orton, CG. High-dose-rate brachytherapy may be radiobiologically superior to low-dose rate due to slow repair of late-responding normal tissue cells. *Int J Radiat Oncol Biol Phys.*, 2001, 49, 183-189.

[8]   Patel, FD; Sharma, SC; Negi, PS; Ghoshal, S; Gupta, BD. Low dose rate vs. high dose rate brachytherapy in the treatment of carcinoma of the uterine cervix: a clinical trial. *IntJRadiatOncolBiolPhys.*, 1994, 28, 335-341.

[9]   Wright, J; Jones, G; Whelan, T; Lukka, H. Patient preference for high or low dose rate brachytherapy in carcinoma of the cervix. *RadiotherOncol*, 1994, 33, 187-194.

[10] Pisansky, TM; Gold, DG; Furutani, KM; et al. High-dose-rate brachytherapy in the curative treatment of patients with localized prostate cancer. *Mayo Clin Proc.*, 2008, 83, 1364-1372.

[11] Feder, BH; Syed, AM; Neblett, D. Treatment of extensive carcinoma of the cervix with the "transperineal parametrial butterfly": a prelimary report on the revival of Waterman's approach. *Int J Radiat Oncol Biol Phys.*, 1978, 4, 735-742.

[12] Fleming, P; Nisar Syed, AM; Neblett, D; Puthawala, A; George, FW; 3rd, Townsend, D. Description of an afterloading 192Ir interstitial-intracavitary technique in the treatment of carcinoma of the vagina. *Obstet Gynecol, 1980*, 55, 525-530.

[13] Aristizabal, SA; Surwit, EA; Hevezi, JM; Heusinkveld, RS. Treatment of advanced cancer of the cervix with transperineal interstitial irradiation. *Int J Radiat Oncol Biol Phys.*, 1983, 9, 1013-1017.

[14] Stock, RG; Chan, K; Terk, M; Dewyngaert, JK; Stone, NN; Dottino, P. A new technique for performing Syed-Neblett template interstitial implants for gynecologic malignancies using transrectal-ultrasound guidance. *IntJRadiatOncolBiolPhys.*, 1997, 37, 819-825.

[15] Nag, S; Martinez-Monge, R; Ellis, R; et al. The use of fluoroscopy to guide needle placement in interstitial gynecological brachytherapy. *Int J Radiat Oncol Biol Phys.*, 1998, 40, 415-420.

[16] Lessard, E; Hsu, IC; Pouliot, J. Inverse planning for interstitial gynecologic template brachytherapy: truly anatomy-based planning. *Int J Radiat Oncol Biol Phys.*, 2002, 54, 1243-1251.

[17] Potter, R; Haie-Meder, C; Van Limbergen, E; et al. Recommendations from gynaecological (GYN) GEC ESTRO working group (II): concepts and terms in 3D image-based treatment planning in cervix cancer brachytherapy-3D dose volume parameters and aspects of 3D image-based anatomy, radiation physics, radiobiology. *Radiother Oncol*, 2006, 78, 67-77.

[18] Wu, A; Ulin, K; Sternick, ES. A dose homogeneity index for evaluating 192Ir interstitial breast implants. *MedPhys.*, 1988, 15, 104-107.

[19] Nag, S; Gupta, N. A simple method of obtaining equivalent doses for use in HDR brachytherapy. *IntJRadiatOncolBiolPhys.*, 2000, 46, 507-513.

[20] Nag, S; Chao, C; Erickson, B; et al. The American Brachytherapy Society recommendations for low-dose-rate brachytherapy for carcinoma of the cervix. *IntJRadiatOncolBiolPhys.*, 2002, 52, 33-48.

[21] Kim, SH; Choi, BI; Lee, HP; et al. Uterine cervical carcinoma: comparison of CT and MR findings. *Radiology*, 1990, 175, 45-51.

[22] Nag, S; Cardenes, H; Chang, S; et al. Proposed guidelines for image-based intracavitary brachytherapy for cervical carcinoma: report from Image-Guided Brachytherapy Working Group. *Int J Radiat Oncol Biol Phys.*, 2004, 60, 1160-1172.

[23] Demanes, DJ; Rodriguez, RR; Bendre, DD; Ewing, TL. High dose rate transperineal interstitial brachytherapy for cervical cancer, high pelvic control and low complication rates. *Int J Radiat Oncol Biol Phys.*, 1999, 45, 105-112.

[24] Itami, J; Hara, R; Kozuka, T; et al. Transperineal high-dose-rate interstitial radiation therapy in the management of gynecologic malignancies. *Strahlenther Onkol*, 2003, 179, 737-741.

[25] Susworo, R; Supriana, N; Ramli, I. HDR interstitial perineal implant for locally advanced or recurrent uterine cervix cancer. *Radiat Med*, 2004, 22, 2-5.

[26] Sitathanee, C; Pairatchvet, V; Narkwong, L; Puataweepong, P. High-dose-rate interstitial brachytherapy in the management of carcinoma of the uterine cervix and other gynecologic malignancies. *JMedAssocThai*, 2005, 88, 1045-1050.

[27] Beriwal, S; Bhatnagar, A; Heron, DE; et al. High-dose-rate interstitial brachytherapy for gynecologic malignancies. *Brachytherapy*, 2006, 5, 218-222.

[28] Viswanathan, AN; Cormack, R; Holloway, CL; et al. Magnetic resonance-guided interstitial therapy for vaginal recurrence of endometrial cancer. *IntJRadiatOncolBiolPhys.*, 2006, 66, 91-99.

[29] Nandwani, PK; Vyas, RK; Neema, JP; Suryanarayan, UK; Bhavsar, DC; Jani, KR. Retrospective analysis of role of interstitial brachytherapy using template (MUPIT) in locally advanced gynecological malignancies. *JCancerResTher.*, 2007, 3, 111-115.

[30] Badakh, DK; Grover, AH. Reirradiation with high-dose-rate remote afterloading brachytherapy implant in patients with locally recurrent or residual cervical carcinoma. *JCancerResTher.*, 2009, 5, 24-30.

[31] Isohashi, F; Yoshioka, Y; Koizumi, M; et al. High-dose-rate interstitial brachytherapy for previously untreated cervical carcinoma. *Brachytherapy*, 2009, 8, 234-239.

[32] Yoshida, K; Yamazaki, H; Takenaka, T; et al. A Dose-Volume Analysis of Magnetic Resonance Imaging-Aided High-Dose-Rate Image-Based Interstitial Brachytherapy for Uterine Cervical Cancer. *Int J Radiat Oncol Biol Phys.*, 2009.

[33] Kushner, DM; Fleming, PA; Kennedy, AW; Wilkinson, DA; Lee, E; Saffle, PA. High dose rate (192)Ir afterloading brachytherapy for cancer of the vagina. *BrJRadiol*, 2003, 76, 719-725.

[34] Beriwal, S; Heron, DE; Mogus, R; Edwards, RP; Kelley, JL; Sukumvanich, P. High-dose rate brachytherapy (HDRB) for primary or recurrent cancer in the vagina. *RadiatOncol*, 2008, 3, 7.

[35] Shah, AP; Strauss, JB; Gielda, BT; Zusag, TW. Toxicity Associated with Bowel or Bladder Puncture During Gynecologic Interstitial Brachytherapy. *IntJRadiatOncolBiolPhys.*, 2009.

[36] Kim, DH; Wang-Chesebro, A; Weinberg, V; et al. High-dose rate brachytherapy using inverse planning simulated annealing for locoregionally advanced cervical cancer: a clinical report with 2-year follow-up. *Int J Radiat Oncol Biol Phys.*, 2009, 75, 1329-1334.

[37] Hughes-Davies, L; Silver, B; Kapp, DS. Parametrial interstitial brachytherapy for advanced or recurrent pelvic malignancy: the Harvard/Stanford experience. *GynecolOncol*, 1995, 58, 24-27.

[38] Monk, BJ; Tewari, K; Burger, RA; Johnson, MT; Montz, FJ; Berman, ML. A comparison of intracavitary versus interstitial irradiation in the treatment of cervical cancer. *GynecolOncol*, 1997, 67, 241-247.

[39] Charra, C; Roy, P; Coquard, R; Romestaing, P; Ardiet, JM; Gerard, JP. Outcome of treatment of upper third vaginal recurrences of cervical and endometrial carcinomas with interstitial brachytherapy. *Int J Radiat Oncol Biol Phys.*, 1998, 40, 421-426.

[40] Gupta, AK; Vicini, FA; Frazier, AJ; et al. Iridium-192 transperineal interstitial brachytherapy for locally advanced or recurrent gynecological malignancies. *Int J Radiat Oncol Biol Phys.*, 1999, 43, 1055-1060.

[41] Tewari, K; Cappuccini, F; Brewster, WR; et al. Interstitial brachytherapy for vaginal recurrences of endometrial carcinoma. *Gynecol Oncol*, 1999, 74, 416-422.

[42] Tewari, KS; Cappuccini, F; Puthawala, AA; et al. Primary invasive carcinoma of the vagina: treatment with interstitial brachytherapy. *Cancer*, 2001, 91, 758-770.

[43] Nag, S; Yacoub, S; Copeland, LJ; Fowler, JM. Interstitial brachytherapy for salvage treatment of vaginal recurrences in previously unirradiated endometrial cancer patients. *IntJRadiatOncolBiolPhys.*, 2002, 54, 1153-1159.

[44] Syed, AM; Puthawala, AA; Abdelaziz, NN; et al. Long-term results of low-dose-rate interstitial-intracavitary brachytherapy in the treatment of carcinoma of the cervix. *Int J Radiat Oncol Biol Phys.*, 2002, 54, 67-78.

[45] Dimopoulos, JC; Lang, S; Kirisits, C; et al. Dose-volume histogram parameters and local tumor control in magnetic resonance image-guided cervical cancer brachytherapy. *Int J Radiat Oncol Biol Phys.*, 2009, 75, 56-63.

[46] Dimopoulos, JC; Potter, R; Lang, S; et al. Dose-effect relationship for local control of cervical cancer by magnetic resonance image-guided brachytherapy. *Radiother Oncol*, 2009, 93, 311-315.

[47] Ampuero, F; Doss, LL; Khan, M; Skipper, B; Hilgers, RD. The Syed-Neblett interstitial template in locally advanced gynecological malignancies. *Int J Radiat Oncol Biol Phys.*, 1983, 9, 1897-1903.

[48] Faria, SL; Souhami, L; Joshua, B; Vuong, T; Freeman, CR. Reporting late rectal toxicity in prostate cancer patients treated with curative radiation treatment. *Int J Radiat Oncol Biol Phys.*, 2008, 72, 777-781.

[49] Viswanathan, AN; Dimopoulos, J; Kirisits, C; Berger, D; Potter, R. Computed tomography versus magnetic resonance imaging-based contouring in cervical cancer brachytherapy: results of a prospective trial and preliminary guidelines for standardized contours. *Int J Radiat Oncol Biol Phys.*, 2007, 68, 491-498.

[50] Wachter-Gerstner, N; Wachter, S; Reinstadler, E; et al. Bladder and rectum dose defined from MRI based treatment planning for cervix cancer brachytherapy: comparison of dose-volume histograms for organ contours and organ wall, comparison with ICRU rectum and bladder reference point. *RadiotherOncol*, 2003, 68, 269-276.

[51] Lang, S; Nulens, A; Briot, E; et al. Intercomparison of treatment concepts for MR image assisted brachytherapy of cervical carcinoma based on GYN GEC-ESTRO recommendations. *Radiother Oncol*, 2006, 78, 185-193.

[52] Koom, WS; Sohn, DK; Kim, JY; et al. Computed tomography-based high-dose-rate intracavitary brachytherapy for uterine cervical cancer: preliminary demonstration of correlation between dose-volume parameters and rectal mucosal changes observed by flexible sigmoidoscopy. *Int J Radiat Oncol Biol Phys.*, 2007, 68, 1446-1454.

[53] Beriwal, S; Kim, H; Coon, D; et al. Single magnetic resonance imaging vs magnetic resonance imaging/computed tomography planning in cervical cancer brachytherapy. *Clin Oncol (R Coll Radiol)* 2009, 21, 483-487.

[54] Kubicky, CD; Yeh, BM; Lessard, E; et al. Inverse planning simulated annealing for magnetic resonance imaging-based intracavitary high-dose-rate brachytherapy for cervical cancer. *Brachytherapy*, 2008, 7, 242-247.

[55] Georg, P; Kirisits, C; Goldner, G; et al. Correlation of dose-volume parameters, endoscopic and clinical rectal side effects in cervix cancer patients treated with definitive radiotherapy including MRI-based brachytherapy. *RadiotherOncol*, 2009, 91, 173-180.

[56] Yaparpalvi, R; Mutyala, S; Gorla, GR; et al. Point vs. volumetric bladder and rectal doses in combined intracavitary-interstitial high-dose-rate brachytherapy: correlation and comparison with published Vienna applicator data. *Brachytherapy*, 2008, 7, 336-342.

[57] Haie-Meder, C; Dumas, I; Paumier, A; et al. [Implementation of GEC-ESTRO recommendations on 3-D based image brachytherapy]. *CancerRadiother*, 2008, 12, 522-526.

[58] Kirisits, C; Potter, R; Lang, S; Dimopoulos, J; Wachter-Gerstner, N; Georg, D. Dose and volume parameters for MRI-based treatment planning in intracavitary brachytherapy for cervical cancer. *IntJRadiatOncolBiolPhys.*, 2005, 62, 901-911.

[59] Kovacs, G; Potter, R; Loch, T; et al. GEC/ESTRO-EAU recommendations on temporary brachytherapy using stepping sources for localised prostate cancer. *RadiotherOncol*, 2005, 74, 137-148.

[60] Salembier, C; Lavagnini, P; Nickers, P; et al. Tumour and target volumes in permanent prostate brachytherapy: a supplement to the ESTRO/EAU/EORTC recommendations on prostate brachytherapy. *RadiotherOncol*, 2007, 83, 3-10.

[61] Akimoto, T; Ito, K; Saitoh, J; et al. Acute genitourinary toxicity after high-dose-rate (HDR) brachytherapy combined with hypofractionated external-beam radiation therapy for localized prostate cancer: correlation between the urethral dose in HDR brachytherapy and the severity of acute genitourinary toxicity. *IntJRadiat OncolBiolPhys.*, 2005, 63, 463-471.

[62] Akimoto, T; Katoh, H; Noda, SE; et al. Acute genitourinary toxicity after high dose rate (HDR) brachytherapy combined with hypofractionated external-beam radiation therapy for localized prostate cancer: Second analysis to determine the correlation between the urethral dose in HDR brachytherapy and the severity of acute genitourinary toxicity. *Int J Radiat Oncol Biol Phys.*, 2005, 63, 472-478.

[63] Nose, T; Koizumi, M; Yoshida, K; et al. In vivo dosimetry of high-dose-rate interstitial brachytherapy in the pelvic region: use of a radiophotoluminescence glass dosimeter for measurement of 1004 points in 66 patients with pelvic malignancy. *IntJRadiat OncolBiolPhys.*, 2008, 70, 626-633.

In: Brachytherapy
Editor: Leoni M. Fischer

ISBN: 978-1-61728-750-3
© 2011 Nova Science Publishers, Inc.

Chapter 3

High-Dose-Rate (HDR) Intracavitary Brachytherapy (ICBT) for Cervical Cancer: Advances for Better Local Control and Complications Sparing

Eng-Yen Huang*

Department of Radiation Oncology,Chang Gung Memorial Hospital-Kaohsiung Medical Center, Chang Gung University, Taiwan

Abstract

High-dose-rate (HDR) intracavitary brachytherapy (ICBT) is widely applied for patients with cervical cancer. The advantages of HDR-ICBT are time and resource conservation, outpatient service, convenience, and optimal cost-effectiveness. Meta-analysis shows similar local control and complications in comparison with low dose rate ICBT. The rectum is the most common organ at risk (OAR) in the reports about HDR-ICBT. The International Commission on Radiation Units and Measurements (ICRU) 38 report defined reference points for dosimetry. The rectal complications are related not only to cumulative ICRU doses to the rectum, but also to external parametrial doses (PMD). For diminishing biologically effective dose (BED) of the rectum, rectal balloon inflation, small fraction size of point A, or intensity modulated radiation therapy (IMRT) may be beneficial to patients with potentially high rectal doses. Correlations between dosimetry and complications of the urinary bladder and sigmoid colon are controversial due to organ movement. CT/MRI-based treatment planning is suggested for more accurate dosimetry because doses of ICRU reference points are typically underestimated using orthogonal radiography-based dosimetry. To improve local control rate, MRI-guided brachytherapy is preferred for better target delineation and dose coverage. The unsolved issues of HDR-ICBT are weighting relative to external beam radiation therapy, dose rate effect, impact of concurrent chemotherapy, optimal dose-fraction, interfractional dose variation, brachytherapy devices, dosimetry using 3D planning, and

---

* Corresponding author: E-mail: huangengyen@gmail.com

reference points/volume for OAR. This chapter presents a comprehensive literature review and discussion.

Introduction

High-dose-rate (HDR) intracavitary brachytherapy (ICBT) is widely practiced for patients with cervical cancer.The HDR technique accounts for 100%, 89%, 50~70%, and 13.3% of ICBT in Taiwan, Japan (Toita 2009), Europe (Guedea et al. 2007), and the United States (Erickson et al. 2005), respectively. In Canada, the dose rate of ICBT is currently changing to an HDR technique (Pearce et al. 2009). The source and applicator of HDR-ICBT are smaller than LDR-ICBT. HDR-ICBT also allows for shorter treatment time and causes less patient discomfort. Patient activity is not limited after applicator removal and the next patient can be immediately treated. HDR-ICBT is suitable for a large number of patients and is cost-effective. Due to several HDR-ICBT experiencesrelated to local control and complications, the following issues need to be clarified and discussed.

Dose Rate Effect

Low dose rate (LDR) intracavitary brachytherapy may have the advantage of fewer complications because it allows for sublethal damage repair (Stewart et al. 2006).However, meta-analysis shows no differences between HDR and LDR for overall survival, local recurrence and late complications (Viani et al. 2009).The comparisons of differences of source, applicator, and fractionations used in brachytherapy are controversial (Stewart et al. 2006). The optimal adjustment of dose rate effect must be compared by the same source and applicator use. Hence, source activity partially represents dose rate. Suzuki et al. first reported the dose-rate effect of HDR ^{192}Ir on late rectal bleeding in patients (n=132) undergoing HDR-ICBT (Suzuki et al. 2008). This suggests that when source activity is higher than 2.4 $cGy \cdot m^2 \cdot h^{-1}$, ICBT should be performed with more caution not to exceed 100 Gy_3 in total. According to the study of Suzuki et al., dose rate effect may exist in patients whose cumulative rectal biologically effective dose(CRBED) exceeds 100 Gy_3. However, source activity cannot be modified when the patient is appointed to undergo ICBT. Waiting for source activity to decay below 2.4 $cGy \cdot m^2 \cdot h^{-1}$ is impossible because total treatment time will be prolonged. Hence, sufficient vaginal packing should reduce the rectal dose. Decreasing the dose rate in the rectum and controlling the CRBED below 100 Gy_3 is also possible. In another study, Kim et al. failed to prove the dose rate effect of rectal and bladder complications (Kim et al. 2008). The sample size was too small (n=54) to detect the difference. Dose rate effect may exist in certain subgroups (e.g., high cumulative BED, high external beam dose).

Fraction Size

According to the concept of radiobiology, large fraction size has a large biologically effective dose (BED) if the α/β ratio of normal tissue is 3. Applying conventional daily radiotherapy in brachytherapy is typically used to estimate BED of organ at risk (OAR). Studying the effect of fraction size from a single institute may be easy to perform because of consistent EBRT dose and similar patient population. However, the sample size should be large enough to detect a statistical difference and a long-term follow-up after the study is time consuming. Hence, the number of studies is limited. Although few studies compare treatment outcomes of different fractionation schedules, the following evidence favors using a small fraction size to reduce complication without compromising tumor control.

Our retrospective study (7.2 Gy for 3 fractions versus 4.8 Gy for 5 fractions) revealed more low-grade rectal complications in patients undergoing a large fraction size of HDR-ICBT (Wang et al. 2004).Our recent prospective cohort study that compares two fractionation schedules (6 Gy for 4 fractions versus 4.5 Gy for 6 fractions) also confirmed this concept in patients with age > 63 years (unpublished data). Larger fraction size has an impact on $\geq$ Grade 2 but not $\geq$ Grade 3 proctitis. The difference between recent and prior studies is a lower parametrial dose (PMD) in the recent study. Hsu et al. compared two fractionation schedules (8 Gy for 4 fractions versus 7 Gy for 6 fractions) and noted more complications in 7 Gy for 6 fractions (Hsu et al. 1995). However, the estimated BED of 7 Gy $\times$ 6 and is 8 Gy $\times$ 4 is 140 Gy_3 and 117 Gy_3, respectively. Although the ICRU rectal point dose is expected to be lower than the point A dose, the CRBED is high following the summation by BED of EBRT. It is reasonable to explain the high complication rate in the 7 Gy $\times$ 6 scheme due to high BED twice per day. Orton et al. suggested a fraction size < 7 Gy to avoid severe or moderate plus severe complications (Orton et al. 1991). Clark et al. suggested that a reduced fraction size from 10 Gy to 8 Gy for 3 fractions to achieve CRBED < 125 Gy_3 following EBRT 46 Gy (Clark et al. 1997).

Chatani et al. conducted a prospective randomized study (n=165) and compared two fractionation schedules (6 Gy vs. 7.5 Gy) (Chatani et al. 1994). No statistically significant differences were noted between the two treatment schedules in survival rates, failure patterns and complications rates. Wong et al. compared two fractionation schedules (6 Gy $\times$ 4 vs. 7 Gy $\times$ 3) (n=220) and also noted no significant differences of local control and complications rates (Wong et al. 2003). They showed a statistical trend (p=0.0672) for the five-year overall complication rate (44.2%) of the four-fraction regimen compared to that of the three-fraction regimen (55.8%). According to the above studies, an appropriate choice of small fraction size may reduce complications and maintain tumor control, especially in elderly patients. Further studies of fraction size could identify which schedule is suitable for certain groups of patients. A department could choose different dose schedules for individualized treatment.

Cumulative Rectal Biologically Effective Dose (CRBED)

Rectal complications are not only caused by the ICBT dose, but also by the external beam dose. The analysis is complex because of the discord between EBRT and ICBT. Hence, CRBED is used to integrate from the physical to the biological dose. Some studies have revealed a positive correlation between CRBED and rectal complications (Table 1). The threshold dose varies from 100 to 147 Gy_3, depending on the grade of rectal complications. Ogino et al. reported 253 patients undergoing either 5-6 Gy × 5-6 fractions or 3.75 Gy × 8 fractions to point A (Ogino et al. 1995). They found a similar mean CRBED between the two dose schedules: Grade 0-4: 147.8 Gy_3 versus 146.6 Gy_3; Grade 1-4: 167.4 Gy_3 versus 164.5 Gy_3; Grade 3-4: 182.1 Gy3 versus 174.1 Gy_3, seen in the dose-response relationship in CRBED and the grade. Grade 4 rectal complication was not observed in any patients with CRBED < 147 Gy_3. Clark et al. estimated the threshold of rectal complications as CRBED < 125 Gy_3 (Clarket al. 1997).

We first identified the effect of CRBED that is dependent on externalPMD. CRBED > 100 Gy_3 is associated with severe proctitis in patients whose external PMD is 54 Gy or greater but not < 54 Gy (Huang et al. 2004). Suzuki et al. also used 100 Gy_3 for correlating rectal bleeding when source activity is higher than 2.4 $cGy \cdot m^2 \cdot h^{-1}$ (Suzuki et al. 2008). The disagreement of CRBED for rectal complications may be related to the above conditions, such as PMD (Huang et al. 2004) and source activity(Suzuki 2008). Chen et al. introduced a geometrical sparing factor (GSF) (i.e. ratio of rectal or bladder dose to point A) and noted that high GSF was associated with rectal and bladder complications (Chen et al. 2009). This concept is similar to their previous study about CRBED (Chen et al. 2000). I believe that patients with high GSF of the rectum correlate with high CRBED. The predictive factors of rectal complications in the study of Chen et al. were at the advanced stage (IIB or greater), age > 70, and CRD > 65 Gy (Chen et al. 2000). Their PMD was 54-58 Gy in advanced-stage patients (77%). The effect of high PMD in the advanced stage confirms our analysis for rectal complications (Huang et al. 2000, 2004). The total rectal dose is expected to be 21-24 Gy/3-4 fractions in patients with CRD > 65 Gy. I predict high CRBED and GSF in their study. Age is an important factor associated with rectal dose in our recent study (Huang et al. 2010). Age and an advanced stage may be partially translated to a high rectal dose (CRD/CRBED) and high PMD, respectively. Significant effects of PMD in our study (Huang et al. 2000) and the age/stage (Chen et al. 2000) in their prior study on rectal complications do not exist in their further studies (Chen et al. 2004, 2009). This may be related to introducing bladder complications as a covariate that is a post-treatment factor misapplied for predicting rectal complications.

Some studies have shown that CRBED is not important. The sample size and PMD must be considered during interpretation. Lee et al. reported a lack of association between CRBED and rectal complications in patients with Stage IB (Lee et al. 2002). Low PMD were delivered to patients due to Stage IB. No Grade 3-4 rectal or bladder complications were noted. Ferrigno et al. also noted no correlation between rectal or bladder complications and cumulative biologic effective dose (Ferrigno et al. 2001). The median dose of the parametrial boost following 45 Gy whole pelvic irradiation was 14.4 Gy.

Table 1. Literature review of association between cumulative rectal biologically effective dose (CRBED) and rectal complications

Authors, year, patient number	PMD (Gy)	CRBED Cutoff	Complication rate
Chen et al.2000 (n=128)	44-59 (median 58)	110 Gy_3*	19.6% vs. 36.4% (crude)
Toita et al. 2003 (n=88)	50	100 Gy_3	4% vs. 31% (3-year)
Chun et al. 2004 (n=268)	45-53	100 Gy_3*	4.2% vs. 19.7% (crude)
Huang et al.2004 (n=297)	39.6-61.2 (median 54)	100 Gy_3*	4% vs. 11% (5-year) (Grade 3-4)
Hyun Kim et al. 2005 (n=157)	41.4-66	125 Gy_3*	5.4% vs. 36.1% (5-year) (Grade 2-4)
Noda et al. 2007 (n=92)	49.8-60.6	140 Gy_3*#	13.6% vs. 48.5% (crude)
Suzuki et al. 2008 (n=132)	40-60 (median 50)	100 Gy_3	18% vs. 46% (3-year)

Abbreviation: MVA= multivariate analysis; PMD= parametrial dose
* Multivariate analysis was performed.
# CT-based dosimetry

Hence, the PMD is high. The five-year rectal complication rates were 12% and 18% (p = 0.49) in patients whose BED < 110 Gy_3 and > 110 Gy_3, respectively. The five-year bladder complication rates were 9% and 17% (p = 0.27) in patients whose BED were < 125 Gy_3 and > 125 Gy_3, respectively. Although there was no statistical difference in complication rates between low BED and high BED, we thought the sample size was too low (n= 138) to detect the difference. Another example of CRBED failure to predict rectal complications is noted in the study of Kim et al. (Kim et al. 2008) that reported five-year rectal complications of 33% and 67% (p=0.48) in patients whose BED were < 135 Gy_3 and > 135 Gy_3. The five-year bladder complications of 8% and 33% (p=0.005) were in patients whose cumulative bladder BED were < 130 Gy_3 and > 130 Gy_3, respectively. Multivariate analysis also showed a comparable result with univariate analysis. The sample size was fifty-four patients and the median PMD was 50.4 Gy.

The most criticism of CRBED as a predictor is that ICRU rectal dose is only a point dose. The ICRU rectal point is inadequate to present the rectum volume correlated to rectal complications. To answer the question, CT-based dosimetry should be used to compare and correlate the dose of ICRU reference point and the dose of OAR volume. Wang et al. failed to strongly correlate the dose of ICRU rectal point with the dose of rectal volume such as D(RV2) (r = 0.251, p = 0.079), D(RV1) (r = 0.279, p = 0.049), and D(BV0.1) (r = 0.282, p = 0.047) (Wang et al. 2009). However, the dose of bladder point strongly correlated to the dose of bladder volume such as D(BV2) (r = 0.668, p < 0.001), D(BV1) (r=0.666, p<0.001), and D(BV0.1) (r = 0.655, p < 0.001). In contrast, Yaparpalvi et al. reported that the ICRU rectal dose correlated with doses of rectal volume $2cm^3$ (r = 0.91, p = 0.0003). No correlation between the ICRU bladder dose and the volumetric bladder dose was noted (Yaparpalvi et al. 2008). Similarly, Pelloski et al. noted no significant difference between the ICRU rectal dose and doses of rectal volume 2 cm^3 (p = 0.561). However, there was a significant difference between the bladder dose and doses of bladder volume 2 cm^3 (p < 0.001) (Pelloski et al. 2005). van den Bergh et al. also noted a high correlation between the ICRU rectal dose and doses of rectal volume 2 cm^3 (r= 0.90) (van den Bergh et al. 1998). Hence, the ICRU rectal point dose may correlate to the dose of rectal volume. If CT/MRI-based dosimetry is not performed, the ICRU rectal point is still important for dose and complication evaluation.

Sigmoid Colon

Few researches have studied the effect of HDR-ICBT on the sigmoid colon until CT/MRI-based dosimetry was applied in treatment planning (Kirisits et al. 2005, Holloway et al. 2009). Kim et al. reported that the mean D3% (dose of 3% volume) for the sigmoid colon dose (3.88 Gy) was higher than the rectum (3.52 Gy) and the small bowel (3.36 Gy) (Kim et al. 2003) when point A dose was 6 Gy. Al-Booz et al. found the sigmoid colon to be a relatively immobile structure (Al-Booz et al. 2006). The dose is usually greater than 70% of the point A dose. Holloway et al. used CT-based dosimetry for evaluating the sigmoid colon dose (Holloway et al. 2009). The distance (median1.7 cm) of the tandem and the sigmoid colon is significantly correlated to the sigmoid dose. Hence, the active length of the tandem may influence the sigmoid dose. Choi et al. noted the impact of anintrauterine tandem length greater than 5 cm on rectoigmoid complications (Choi et al. 1992). However, if active length is too short, poor CTV coverage is notable in the tumor with uterine cavity invasion. MRI-guided ICBT is suggested in patients with uterine cavity invasion for better tumor coverage.

Applicator Position and Type

Applicator positions vary between different fractions in some studies.Wulf et al. noted significant small intrafractonal variability compared to interfractional variability (Wulf et al. 2004). Datta et al. demonstrated that multiple HDR-ICBT applications resulted in significant variation in the applicator geometry and its positions in the pelvis, irrespective of applicator rigidity (Datta et al. 2003). They reported about 0.93-1.51 cm of average displacement at the tandem tip or bilateral ovoid. Grigsby et al. reported that average shift of the vector was 1.0 to 1.5 cm with posterior and inferior displacement (Grigsby et al. 1993).

Does the change of geometry change the dose? Garipağaoğlu et al. used radiography-based dosimetry and reported that the displacement distance is between 2.0 mm and 16.9 mm (Garipağaoğlu et al. 2006). Although the displacement did not significantly affect the rectal and bladder dose, they noted the correlation between rectal dose change and the resultant vector (r = 0.418, p = 0.007). Hoskin et al. found that the change (median10.5 mm) of ICRU rectal point at the second fraction was closer to the ovoid source (Hoskin et al. 1996). However, the confounding factor examination under anesthesia (EUA) allows more vaginal packing at the first fraction. Our previous study also demonstrated that EUA reduces rectal dose (Huang et al. 2010). Elhanafy et al. also used vector analysis and revealed that the magnitude of the average shift ranged from 10-13 mm (Elhanafy et al. 2002). A dose difference of >20% for the bladder and rectum points, but < than 8% for the other points was noted. Pham et al. found anterior shifts correlating with high bladder dose differences of 17.4% (Pham et al. 1998). Davidson et al. used CT-based dosimetry and found significant increases to the rectal dose at 2 cm^3 if a single plan is used for an entire course of HDR-ICBT

(Davidson et al. 2008). They also analyzed the effect of applicator-specific results and revealed a significant increase ($p< 0.030$) to dose points and volumes for the rectum and bladder for tandem-ring (TO) applicators. Conversely, dose values from tandem-ovoids (TR) did not show any significant trend. Chi et al. also reported similar results of increased dose to 2 cm^3 of OARs with the single plan (Chi et al. 2009). The dose variation was statistically similar between the TO and TR groups. Levin et al. also found no significant differences between TO and TR applicators in doses to point A, ICRU bladder point, or 2 cm^3 of OARs (Levin 2008). However, doses of point B and ICRU rectal point and treatment volumes/time were higher in TO than TR.

In addition to applicator geometry, the effect of vaginal packing on rectal and bladder dose is also important in each fraction because these doses are sensitive to the extent of packing. Kim et al. noted that vaginal packing in the first fraction (41%) was better than in the last fraction (0%) in patients receiving conscious sedation (Kim et al. 1995). Taken together, interfractional dose variations exist and dosimetric planning at each fraction is favored.

Table 2. The American Brachytherapy Society suggestions in doses of EBRT and HDR-ICBT for cervical cancer

EBRT doses (Gy)	HDR dose (Gy) per fraction	Fractions	LQED2	Total LQED2
Early stage				
20	7.5	6	65.6	85.6
20	6.5	7	62.6	82.6
20	6	8	64	84
45	6	5	40	85
45	5.3	6	40.6	85.6
Advanced stage				
45	6.5	5	44.6	89.6
45	5.8	6	45.8	90.8
50.4	7	4	39.7	90.1
50.4	6	5	40	90.4
50.4	5.3	6	40.6	91

Abbreviation: HDR= high dose rate; ICBT= intracavitary bachytherapy; EBRT = external beam radiation therapy; LQED2= linear quadratic equivalent dose for a 2 Gy fraction
Total LQED2 = EBRT dose + LQED2

Weighting of EBRT and ICBT

The American Brachytherapy Society (ABS) recommends weighting EBRT and HDR-ICBT for carcinoma of the cervix (Table 2) (Nag et al. 2000). The EBRT dose should be limited to 45 Gy and 50.4 Gy in the early and advanced stage, respectively. The suggested fractions and fraction size in the early stage is 6-8 fractions and 5.3-7.5 Gy dependent on the EBRT dose. The suggested fractions and fraction size in the advanced stage are 4-6 fractions and 5.3-7 Gy dependent on the EBRT dose. Logsdon et al. reported treatment outcomes in 907 stage IIIB patients without systemic concurrent chemotherapy (Logsdon et al. 1999). They suggested combining 40-45 Gy of EBRT with more intensive ICBT to achieve the highest five-year disease-free survival (DSS) rates (53%) and the lowest major complication rates (15%). Although they used LDR-ICBT, the effect of HDR-ICBT is equal to LDR-ICBT in meta-analysis (Viani et al. 2009). After 1999, CCRT has been the standard therapy for locally advanced cervical cancer and CCRT enhances local control (Morris et al. 1999). The suggestion can also be followed in patients with HDR-ICBT.

Chemotherapy

Few studies have demonstrated the positive impact of concurrent chemoradiotherapy (CCRT) on late complications. Clark et al. reported the impact of CCRT on late rectal complications and estimated that the probability increased in patients with weekly cisplatin while CRBED was high (about 200-250 Gy_3) (Clarket al. 1997). Rakovitch et al. noted that mitomycin C increased late bowel obstruction and rectum accounted for about one half of complications (Rakovitch et al. 1997). The EBRT doses ranged from 45-52.8 Gy. Many studies reporting patients undergoing HDR-ICBT with or without chemotherapy did not show chemotherapy as an adverse factor in late complications. Hence, there is no strong evidence showing that CCRT increases rectal or bladder complications in patients with HDR-ICBT. However, chemotherapy-induced hematological and gastrointestinal toxicities may result in discomfort during ICBT application. A complete blood count is suggested before application.

Effect of Bladder and Rectal Distension

Studies have shown no evidence of a correlation between doses to the ICRU reference bladder point and bladder complications in patients undergoing HDR-ICBT. Toita et al. did not find a correlation with incidence and severity (Toita et al. 2003). The reasons for a lack of positive correlation are as follows. The onset of bladder complications occur later than rectal complications. It needs much more follow-up timeto study the bladder complications. The ICRU bladder point is located at the bladder neck. Similar to the rectum, a point dose does not present the volume of the whole organ. Furthermore, the position of the Foley catheter balloon may vary. Bladder volume is also variable. Hence, CT/MRI-assisted planning improves accuracy of the bladder dose evaluation.

Based on the concept of bladder fullness to decrease small-bowel volume irradiated during EBRT, our prior study evaluated the effect of HDR-ICBT (Sunet al. 2005). We noted that bladder distension statistically significantly decreased the median bladder wall dose with an average reduction of 48% of the dose of an empty bladder ($p< 0.001$). Cengiz et al. demonstrated that bladder distension decreased the median maximum dose of the small bowel and bladder from 4.93 to 2.84 Gy and from 9.93 to 9.25 Gy, respectively. The median maximum dose of the rectum also decreased from 6.28 to 4.81 Gy (Cengiz et al. 2008). Kim et al. also evaluated the effect of bladder distension on dosimetry of OARs (Kim et al. 2010). They found that bladder distension decreased the small-bowel dose (D 2cc) from 4.75 to 2.16

Gy ($p<$ 0.001). The mean dose of 50% volume (D50%) of the small bowel and bladder also decreased from 2.82 to 2.21 Gy (p = 0.004) and from 1.08 to 0.80 Gy ($p<$ 0.001), respectively. According to the above studies, bladder distension has a beneficial effect on OARs.

No strong evidence exists regarding rectal inflation reducing rectal dose during HDR-ICBT for cervical cancer. The concept for prostate cancer 3DCRT/IMRT is well applied. Teh et al. reported that using a rectal balloon could not only immobilize the prostate, but also reduce the rectal wall dose in patients with prostate cancer undergoing IMRT (Teh et al. 2002, 2005). Patel et al. also demonstrated that (Patel et al. 2003) using an endorectal balloon with a 3D-CRT plan produced about as much rectal dose sparing. van Lin et al. reported that rectal balloon reduced late rectal complication (van Lin et al. 2007). Whether rectal inflation can reduce the rectal dose of ICBT needs further investigation.

CT/MRI-Assisted Treatment Planning

The GEC-ESTRO working group recommended clear descriptions of GTV_D (at diagnosis), CTV_D, GTV_B (at brachytherapy), CTV_B, high risk (HR) CTV (residual macroscopic disease), and intermediate risk (IR) CTV (residual macroscopic plus microscopic disease) in MRI-based dosimetry (Haie-Meder et al. 2005). The GEC-ESTRO working group (Pötter et al. 2006)also suggested a report of the 3D image-basedDVH parameters for GTV, HR CTV and IR CTV with the minimum dose delivered to 90% (D90) and 100% (D100) of volume. The volumeof the prescribed dose 100% (V100), 150% (V150) and 200% (V200) is also recommended. V100 is recommended for quality assessment only within a given treatment schedule. The minimum doses in the OARat 0.1, 1, and 2 cm^3 are required for reporting.

An increasing number of studies have discussed CT/MRI-based dosimetry that provides clear information of tumor coverage and the dose-volume relationship of OARs. Kim et al. used CT-based dosimetry and noted that the 6 Gy volume encompassed an average GTV of 98.5%, 89.5%, 79.5%, and 59.5% for stages IB1, IB2, IIB, and IIIB, respectively (Kim et al. 2003). The mean dose for the ICRU rectal point and D3% was 3.97 Gy (2.09–5.37) and 3.52 Gy (2.05–4.08), respectively. They reported a dose at 2 cm^3 (D2) of OARs in a further study (Kim 2007). The mean ICRU bladder point dose (4.01Gy) was lower than the mean bladder D2 dose (4.84 Gy). However, the mean ICRU rectal point dose (4.12 Gy) did not differ significantly from the mean rectal D2 dose (3.73 Gy). The most frequent organ receiving the highest D2 dose was the sigmoid colon in nine of twenty-two patients (41%), followed by the rectum in seven of twenty-two patients (32%) and the small bowel in six of twenty-two patients (27%). Onal et al. also noted decreased GTV and CTV coverage with increasing tumor size and stage (Onal et al. 2009). They also found that conventional planning underestimated the ICRU rectal and bladder points dose.Chi et al. conducted a prospective study with customized treatment planning at each fraction of HDR-ICBT (Chi et al. 2009). Applying the initial treatment plan for all other fractions leads to an increased dose to the OARs in general, especially in the bladder. Lang et al. used MRI-assisted planning with total BED constraints for better local control and for minimizing side effects (Lang et al. 2007). These parameters of GEC-ESTRO need further clinical data to validate.

References

Al-Booz, H; Boiangiu, I; Appleby, H; French, C; Coomber, H; Humphery, P; Cornes, P. Sigmoid colon is an unexpected organ at risk in brachytherapy for cervix cancer.*J Egypt Natl Canc Inst.*, 2006, 18(2), 156-60.

Cengiz, M; Gürdalli, S; Selek, U; Yildiz, F; Saglam, Y; Ozyar, E; Atahan, IL. Effect of bladder distension on dose distribution of intracavitary brachytherapy for cervical cancer: three-dimensional computed tomography plan evaluation.*IntJRadiatOncolBiolPhys.*, 2008, 70(2), 464-8.

Chatani, M; Matayoshi, Y; Masaki, N; Teshima, T; Inoue, T. A prospective randomized study concerning the point A dose in high-dose rate intracavitary therapy for carcinoma of the uterine cervix. The final results. *Strahlenther Onkol*, 1994, 170(11), 636-42.

Chen, SW; Liang, JA; Yang, SN; Liu, RT; Lin, FJ.The prediction of late rectal complications following the treatment of uterine cervical cancer by high-dose-rate brachytherapy. *IntJRadiatOncolBiolPhys.*, 2000, Jul 1, 47(4), 955-61.

Chen, SW; Liang, JA; Yeh, LS; Yang, SN; Shiau, AC; Lin, FJ. Comparative study of reference points by dosimetric analyses for late complications after uniform external radiotherapy and high-dose-rate brachytherapy for cervical cancer.*IntJRadiatOnco lBiolPhys.*, 2004, 60(2), 663-71.

Chen, SW; Liang, JA; Hung, YC; Yeh, LS; Chang, WC; Yang, SN; Lin, FJ. Geometrical sparing factors for the rectum and bladder in the prediction of grade 2 and higher complications after high-dose-rate brachytherapy for cervical cancer.*IntJRadiat OncolBiolPhys.*, 2009, 75(5), 1335-43.

Chi, A; Gao, M; Sinacore, J; Nguyen, NP; Vali, F; Albuquerque, K. Single versus customized treatment planning for image-guided high-dose-rate brachytherapy for cervical cancer: dosimetric comparison and predicting factor for organs at risk overdose with single plan approach.*Int J Radiat Oncol Biol Phys.*, 2009, 75(1), 309-14.

Choi, P; Teo, P; Foo, W; O, SK; Leung, SF; Tsao, SY; Shiu, W. High-dose-rate remote afterloading irradiation of carcinoma of the cervix in Hong Kong: unexpectedly high complication rate.*Clin Oncol (R Coll Radiol).* 1992, 4(3), 186-91.

Chun, M; Kang, S; Kil, HJ; Oh, YT; Sohn, JH; Ryu, HS. Rectal bleeding and its management after irradiation for uterine cervical cancer.*IntJRadiatOncolBiolPhys.*, 2004, 58(1), 98-105.

Clark, BG; Souhami, L; Roman, TN; Chappell, R; Evans, MD; Fowler, JF. The prediction of late rectal complications in patients treated with high dose-rate brachytherapy for carcinoma of the cervix.*IntJRadiatOncolBiolPhys.*, 1997, 38(5), 989-93.

Datta, NR; Kumar, S; Das, KJ; Pandey, CM; Halder, S; Ayyagari, S. Variations of intracavitary applicator geometry during multiple HDR brachytherapy insertions in carcinoma cervix and its influence on reporting as per ICRU report 38.*Radiother Oncol*, 2001, 60(1), 15-24.

Davidson, MT; Yuen, J; D'Souza, DP; Batchelar, DL. Image-guided cervix high-dose-rate brachytherapy treatment planning: does custom computed tomography planning for each insertion provide better conformal avoidance of organs at risk?*Brachytherapy*, 2008, 7(1), 37-42.

Elhanafy, OA; Das, RK; Paliwal, BR; Migahed, MD; Sakr, HA; Elleithy, M. Anatomic variation of prescription points and treatment volume with fractionated high-dose rate gynecological brachytherapy.*JApplClinMedPhys.*, 2002, 3(1), 1-5.

Erickson, B; Eifel, P; Moughan, J; Rownd, J; Iarocci,T; Owen, J. Patterns of brachytherapy practice for patients with carcinoma of the cervix (1996-1999), a patterns of care study. *Int J Radiat Oncol Biol Phys.*, 2005, 63(4), 1083-92.

Ferrigno, R; dos Santos Novaes, PE; Pellizzon, AC; Maia, MA; Fogarolli, RC; Gentil, AC; Salvajoli, JV. High-dose-rate brachytherapy in the treatment of uterine cervixcancer. Analysis of dose effectiveness and late complications.*IntJRadiatOncolBiolPhys.*, 2001, 50(5), 1123-35.

Garipağaoğlu, M; Tunçel, N; Dalmaz, MG; Gülkesen, H; Toy, A; Kizildağ, AU; Köseoğlu, FG. Changes in applicator positions and dose distribution between high dose rate brachytherapy fractions in cervix carcinoma patients receiving definitive radiotherapy. *Br J Radiol*, 2006, 79(942), 504-9.

Grigsby, PW; Georgiou, A; Williamson, JF; Perez, CA. Anatomic variation of gynecologic brachytherapy prescription points. *IntJRadiatOncolBiolPhys.*, 1993, 27(3), 725-9.

Guedea, F; Ellison, T; Venselaar, J; Borras, JM; Hoskin, P; Poetter, R; Heeren, G; Nisin, R; François, G; Mazeron, JJ; Limbergen, EV; Ventura, M; Taillet, M; Cottier, B. Overview of brachytherapy resources in Europe: a survey of patterns of care study for brachytherapy in Europe. *Radiother Oncol*, 2007, 82(1), 50-4.

Haie-Meder, C; Pötter, R; Van Limbergen, E; Briot, E; De Brabandere, M; Dimopoulos, J; Dumas, I; Hellebust, TP; Kirisits, C; Lang, S; Muschitz, S; Nevinson, J; Nulens, A; Petrow, P; Wachter-Gerstner, N. Gynaecological (GYN) GEC-ESTRO Working Group. Recommendations from Gynaecological (GYN) GEC-ESTRO Working Group (I): concepts and terms in 3D image based 3D treatment planning in cervix cancer brachytherapy with emphasis on MRI assessment of GTV and CTV. *Radiother Oncol.*, 2005, 74(3), 235-45.

Holloway, CL; Racine, ML; Cormack, RA; O'Farrell, DA; Viswanathan, AN. Sigmoid dose using 3D imaging in cervical-cancer brachytherapy. *RadiotherOncol.*, 93(2), 307-10.

Hoskin, PJ; Cook, M; Bouscale, D; Cansdale, J. Changes in applicator position with fractionated high dose rate gynaecological brachytherapy.*Radiother Oncol*, 1996, 40(1), 59-62.

Hsu, WL; Wu, CJ; Jen, YM; Yen, SH; Lin, KT; Ger, LP; Kim, RY. Twice-per-day fractionated high versus continuous low dose rate intracavitary therapy in the radical treatment of cervical cancer: a nonrandomized comparison of treatment results.*Int J Radiat Oncol Biol Phys.*, 1995, 32(5), 1425-31.

Huang, EY; Lin, H; Hsu, HC; Wang, CJ; Chen, HC; Sun, LM; Hsiung, CY. High external parametrial dose can increase the probability of radiation proctitis in patients with uterine cervix cancer. *GynecolOncol*, 2000, 79(3), 406-10.

Huang, EY; Wang, CJ; Hsu, HC; Hao, Lin; Chen, HC; Sun, LM. Dosimetric factors predicting severe radiation-induced bowel complications in patients with cervical cancer: combined effect of external parametrial dose and cumulative rectal dose. *GynecolOncol*, 2004, 95(1), 101-8.

Huang, EY; Wang, CJ; Lan, JH; Chen, HC; Fang, FM; Hsu, HC; Huang, YJ; Wang, CY; Wang, YM. Factors for predicting rectal dose of high-dose-rate intracavitary brachytherapy after pelvic irradiation in patients with cervical cancer: a retrospective study with radiography-based dosimetry.*IntJRadiatOncolBiolPhys.*, 2010, 76(2), 490-5.

Hyun Kim, T; Choi, J; Park, SY; Lee, SH; Lee, KC; Yang, DS; Shin, KH; Cho, KH; Lim, HS; Kim, JY. Dosimetric parameters that predict late rectal complications after curative radiotherapy in patients with uterine cervical carcinoma.*Cancer*, 2005, 104(6), 1304-11.

Kim, RY; Meyer, JT; Plott, WE; Spencer, SA; Meredith, RF; Jennelle, RL; Salter, MM. Major geometric variations between multiple high-dose-rate applications of brachytherapy in cancer of the cervix: frequency and types of variation.*Radiology*, 1995, 195(2), 419-22.

Kim, RY; Pareek, P. Radiography-based treatment planning compared with computed tomography (CT)-based treatment planning for intracavitary brachytherapy in cancer of the cervix: analysis of dose-volume histograms.*Brachytherapy*, 2003, 2(4), 200-6.

Kim, RY; Shen, S; Duan, J.Image-based three-dimensional treatment planning of intracavitary brachytherapy for cancer of the cervix: dose-volume histograms of the bladder, rectum, sigmoid colon, and small bowel. *Brachytherapy*, 2007, 6(3), 187-94.

Kim, HJ; Kim, S; Ha, SW; Wu, HG.Are doses to ICRU reference points valuable for predicting late rectal and bladder morbidity after definitive radiotherapy in uterine cervix cancer?*Tumori*, 2008, 94(3), 327-32.

Kim, RY; Shen, S; Lin, HY; Spencer, SA; De Los Santos, J. Effects of bladder distension on organs at risk in 3D image-based planning of intracavitary brachytherapy for cervical cancer.*IntJRadiatOncolBiolPhys.*, 2010, 76(2), 485-9.

Kirisits, C; Pötter, R; Lang, S; Dimopoulos, J; Wachter-Gerstner, N; Georg, D. Dose and volume parameters for MRI-based treatment planning in intracavitary brachytherapy for cervical cancer.*Int J Radiat Oncol Biol Phys.*, 2005, 62(3), 901-11.

Lang, S; Kirisits, C; Dimopoulos, J; Georg, D; Pötter, R. Treatment planning for MRI assisted brachytherapy of gynecologic malignancies based on total dose constraints.*Int J Radiat Oncol Biol Phys.*, 2007, 69(2), 619-27.

Lee, SW; Suh, CO; Chung, EJ; Kim, GE. Dose optimization of fractionated external radiation and high-dose-rate intracavitary brachytherapy for FIGO stage IB uterine cervical carcinoma.*IntJRadiatOncolBiolPhys.*, 2002, 52(5), 1338-44.

Levin, D; Menhel, J; Rabin, T; Pfeffer, MR; Symon, Z. Dosimetric comparison of tandem and Ovoids vs. tandem and ring for intracavitary gynecologic applications.*Med Dosim*, 2008, 33(4), 315-20.

Logsdon, MD; Eifel, PJ. Figo IIIB squamous cell carcinoma of the cervix: an analysis of prognostic factors emphasizing the balance between external beam and intracavitary radiation therapy.*IntJRadiatOncolBiolPhys.*, 1999, 43(4), 763-75.

Morris, M; Eifel, PJ; Lu, J; Grigsby, PW; Levenback, C; Stevens, RE; Rotman, M; Gershenson, DM; Mutch, DG. Pelvic radiation with concurrent chemotherapy compared with pelvic and para-aortic radiation for high-risk cervical cancer. *N Engl J Med*, 1999, 340, 1137-1143.

Nag, S; Erickson, B; Thomadsen, B; Orton, C; Demanes, JD; Petereit, D. The American Brachytherapy Society recommendations for high-dose-rate brachytherapy for carcinoma of the cervix.*IntJRadiatOncolBiolPhys.*, 2000, 48(1), 201-11.

Noda, SE; Ohno, T; Kato, S; Ishii, T; Saito, O; Wakatsuki, M; Tamaki, T; Watanabe, K; Nakano, T; Tsujii, H. Late rectal complications evaluated by computed tomography-based dose calculations in patients with cervical carcinoma undergoing high-dose-rate brachytherapy.*IntJRadiatOncolBiolPhys.*, 2007, 69(1), 118-24.

Ogino, I; Kitamura, T; Okamoto, N; Yamasita, K; Aikawa, Y; Okajima, H; Matsubara, S. Late rectal complication following high dose rate intracavitary brachytherapy in cancer of the cervix.*IntJRadiatOncolBiolPhys.*, 1995, 31(4), 725-34.

Onal, C; Arslan, G; Topkan, E; Pehlivan, B; Yavuz, M; Oymak, E; Yavuz, A. Comparison of conventional and CT-based planning for intracavitary brachytherapy for cervical cancer: target volume coverage and organs at risk doses.*JExpClinCancerRes..*, 2009, 28, 95.

Orton, CG; Seyedsadr, M; Somnay, A. Comparison of high and low dose rate remote afterloading for cervix cancer and the importance of fractionation.*Int J Radiat Oncol Biol Phys.*, 1991, 21(6), 1425-34.

Patel, RR; Orton, N; Tomé, WA; Chappell, R; Ritter, MA. Rectal dose sparing with a balloon catheter and ultrasound localization in conformal radiation therapy for prostate cancer.*RadiotherOncol*, 2003, 67(3), 285-94.

Pearce, A; Craighead, P; Kay, I; Traptow, L; Doll, C. Brachytherapy for carcinoma of the cervix: a Canadian survey of practice patterns in a changing era. *RadiotherOncol*, 2009, 91(2), 194-6.

Pelloski, CE; Palmer, M; Chronowski, GM; Jhingran, A; Horton, J; Eifel, PJ. Comparison between CT-based volumetric calculations and ICRU reference-point estimates of radiation doses delivered to bladder and rectum during intracavitary radiotherapy for cervical cancer.*IntJRadiatOncolBiolPhys.*, 2005, 62(1), 131-7.

Pham, HT; Chen, Y; Rouby, E; Lustig, RA; Wallner, PE. Changes in high-dose-rate tandem and ovoid applicator positions during treatment in an unfixed brachytherapy system.*Radiology*, 1998, 206(2), 525-31.

Pötter, R; Haie-Meder, C; Van Limbergen, E; Barillot, I; De Brabandere, M; Dimopoulos, J; Dumas, I; Erickson, B; Lang, S; Nulens, A; Petrow, P; Rownd, J; Kirisits, C. GEC ESTRO Working Group. Recommendations from gynaecological (GYN) GEC ESTRO working group (II): concepts and terms in 3D image-based treatment planning in cervix cancer brachytherapy-3D dose volume parameters and aspects of 3D image-based anatomy, radiation physics, radiobiology. *RadiotherOncol*, 2006, 78(1), 67-77.

Rakovitch, E; Fyles, AW; Pintilie, M; Leung, PM. Role of mitomycin C in the development of late bowel toxicity following chemoradiation for locally advanced carcinoma of the cervix.*IntJRadiatOncolBiolPhys.*, 1997, 38(5), 979-87.

Stewart, AJ; Viswanathan, AN. Current controversies in high-dose-rate versus low-dose-rate brachytherapy for cervical cancer. *Cancer*, 2006, 107(5), 908-15.

Sun, LM; Huang, HY; Huang, EY; Wang, CJ; Ko, SF; Lin, H; Song, JC. A prospective study to assess the bladder distension effects on dosimetry in intracavitary brachytherapy of cervical cancer via computed tomography-assisted techniques.*RadiotherOncol*, 2005, 77(1), 77-82.

Suzuki, O; Yoshioka, Y; Isohashi, F; Morimoto, M; Kotsuma, T; Kawaguchi, Y; Konishi, K; Nakamura, S; Shiomi, H; Inoue, T. Effect of high-dose-rate 192Ir source activity on late rectal bleeding after intracavitary radiation therapy for uterine cervix cancer. *IntJRadiatOncolBiolPhys.*, 2008, 71(5), 1329-34.

The, BS; McGary, JE; Dong, L; Mai, WY; Carpenter, LS; Lu, HH; Chiu, JK; Woo, SY; Grant, WH; Butler, EB. The use of rectal balloon during the delivery of intensity modulated radiotherapy (IMRT) for prostate cancer: more than just a prostate gland immobilization device?*CancerJ*, 2002, Nov-Dec, 8(6), 476-83.

Teh, BS; Dong, L; McGary, JE; Mai, WY; Grant, W; 3rd; Butler, EB.Rectal wall sparing by dosimetric effect of rectal balloon used during intensity-modulated radiation therapy (IMRT) for prostate cancer.*MedDosim*, 2005, 30(1), 25-30.

Toita, T; Kakinohana, Y; Ogawa, K; Adachi, G; Moromizato, H; Nagai, Y; Maehama, T; Sakumoto, K; Kanazawa, K; Murayama, S. Combination external beam radiotherapy and high-dose-rate intracavitary brachytherapy for uterine cervical cancer: Analysis of dose and fractionation schedule.*IntJRadiatOncolBiolPhys.*, 2003, 56(5), 1344-53.

Toita, T.Current status and perspectives of brachytherapy for cervical cancer.*Int J Clin Oncol*, 2009, 14(1), 25-30.

van den Bergh, F; Meertens, H; Moonen, L; van Bunningen, B; Blom, A. The use of a transverse CT image for the estimation of the dose given to the rectum in intracavitary brachytherapy for carcinoma of the cervix.*RadiotherOncol*, 1998 Apr, 47(1), 85-90.

van Lin, EN; Kristinsson, J; Philippens, ME; de Jong, DJ; van der Vight, LP; Kaanders, JH; Leer, JW; Visser, AG. Reduced late rectal mucosal changes after prostate three-dimensional conformal radiotherapy with endorectal balloon as observed in repeated endoscopy.*Int J Radiat Oncol Biol Phys.*, 2007, 67(3), 799-811.

Viani, GA; Manta, GB; Stefano, EJ; de Fendi, LI. Brachytherapy for cervix cancer: low-dose rate or high-dose rate brachytherapy - a meta-analysis of clinical trials.*J Exp Clin Cancer Res.*, 2009, 28, 47.

Wang, CJ; Huang, EY; Sun, LM; Chen, HC; Fang, FM; Hsu, HC; Changchien, CC; Leung, SW. Clinical comparison of two linear-quadratic model-based isoeffect fractionation schemes of high-dose-rate intracavitary brachytherapy for cervical cancer. *IntJRadiatOnclBiolPhys.*, 2004, 59(1), 179-89.

Wang, B; Kwon, A; Zhu, Y; Yeo, I; Henson, CF. Image-guided intracavitary high-dose-rate brachytherapy for cervix cancer: A single institutional experience with three-dimensional CT-based planning. *Brachytherapy*, 2009, 8(2), 240-7.

Wong, FC; Tung, SY; Leung, TW; Sze, WK; Wong, VY; Lui, CM; Yuen, KK; O, SK. Treatment results of high-dose-rate remote afterloading brachytherapy for cervical cancer and retrospective comparison of two regimens. *IntJRadiatOncolBiolPhys.*, 2003, 55(5), 1254-64.

Wulf, J; Popp, K; Oppitz, U; Baier, K; Flentje, M. Positional variability of a tandem applicator system in HDR brachytherapy for primary treatment of cervix cancer. Analysis of the anatomic pelvic position and comparison of the applicator positions during five insertions. *Strahlenther Onkol*, 2004, 180(4), 216-24.

Yaparpalvi, R; Mutyala, S; Gorla, GR; Butler, J; Mah, D; Garg, MK; Kalnicki, S. Point vs. volumetric bladder and rectal doses in combined intracavitary-interstitial high-dose-rate brachytherapy: correlation and comparison with published Vienna applicator data.*Brachytherapy*, 2008, 7(4), 336-42.

In: Brachytherapy
Editor: Leoni M. Fische

ISBN: 978-1-61728-750-3
© 2011 Nova Science Publishers, Inc.

Chapter 4

Dermatological Single-Session Beta Emitter Conformational Brachytherapy of Non-Melanocytic Skin Tumours

Antioco F. Sedda[*1], *Cesidio Cipriani*[2]
and Annamaria Carrozzo[3]

[1]Physics and New Materials Dept., ENEA, Rome, Italy.
[2]Nuclear Medicine Dept., S.Eugenio Hospital, Rome, Italy.
[3]Dermatology Dept., Tor Vergata University, Rome, Italy.

Abstract

In the present paper a therapeutic option for the treatment of BasalCell Carcinoma (BCC) and Squamous Cell Carcinoma (SCC) is described. It basically consists in a superficial high dose brachytherapy, characterized by the use of a ready-to-use kit, in which a radioactive beta-emitting isotope, incorporated in a specially formulated inert, synthetic resin, is applied on the surface of BCC and SCC tumours. When the product is applied on the lesion, a beta emitter brachytherapy irradiation is performed, strictly limited to the area and depth affected by the tumour invasion. The electrons from high energy (> 1MeV) beta emitters isotopes deposit more than 90 % of the dose to the first two mm of the skin, which is the depth usually interested from tumour invasion, but spare the deeper tissues from irradiation. The therapy has been used in a large variety of BCC and SCC: tumours of very large sizes, relapsing or recurrent forms, multifocal lesions, without restriction of site, dimension, clinical or histological type, patients clinical situation, with exclusion of the lymphonode metastatic forms. More than 1200 lesions on 370 patients, with histologically, dermoscopically, or clinically confirmed diagnosis of BCC and SCC, have been treated. After a follow up of 12 - 78 months, a complete response was obtained in 98% of the treated lesions, in 89 % of the lesions after a single application, while in 11% of the patients two or three treatments were performed. A clear advantage of the proposed treatment respect to the surgery is especially evident for all the

* Corresponding author: Email: antiocofrancosedda@tiscali.it.

tumours located in difficult sites, on which surgery would be difficult (nose, ears, eyelids, etc.). The technique should be, in our opinion, the first choice treatment in all those patients with a high number of lesions, or with tumour relapses, in those with tumours located in particular sites, where surgery would produce functional mutilations (penis, vulva, eyelids etc.) and, finally, in older, infirm, or otherwise inoperable ones.

Introduction

Non melanocytic skin cancer (NMSC) is the most frequent malignancy among populations of european origin, and in some countries it accounts for about half of all tumours. It comprises basal cell carcinoma (BCC), Bowen's disease, cutaneous squamous cell carcinoma(SCC), and actinic keratosis (AK) (Marks et al1988, Fuet al 2003). During the last decade, worldwide incidence of NMSC has strongly increased, and now represents about 30% of total cancers (Diepgenet al 2002). NMSC occurrence increases with age and its peak is found around the sixth – seventh decade, more frequently in men than in women. Tumours appear very often on sun exposed areas of the body, as the face, neck, bald scalp, hands, shoulders, arms and back; the rim of the ear and the lower lip are especially vulnerable to these cancers. Light-skinned and low-grade phototype individuals are particulaly affected (Armstronget al 2001). Ultraviolet radiation is a major risk factor for NMSC, and cutaneous human papillomavirus is also considered important in playing an active role during the pathogenesis of these cancers(Nindlet al 2007).Among NMSC, BCC is the most common cancer of white populations, and constitutes the 80% of the cases of skin cancer (American Cancer Society 2008, Roewert-Huber et al 2007). Australia has the highest rate of BCC in the world, and certain regions have an incidence of up 2 % per year (Diepgen et al. 2002). BCC is a slow-growing, locally invasive malignant epidermal skin tumour, but metastases are extremely rare (0.03 - 0.6%); they have been described in the subcutaneous tissue, bones, lungs, liver, lymph nodes of the neck. BCC may appear on every region of body skin, but 90% of the lesions appear on the face and the head skin. It is often indolent, and the most frequent variant consists of a superficial, flat pearly-edged patch, which slowly enlarges. The other clinical form are: nodular, nodular-ulcerative, ulcerative (ulcus rodens), sclerodermic and pigmented. The hystopathological peculiar feature shows ingrowths of epidermal keratinocytes adjacent to palisades of cell resembling those that constitute the lower basal layer (Bowden 2004). Evidence suggests that BCC may arise from the pluripotent cells in the basal layer of hair follicles of the skin (Jih 1999).

SCC is the second most common form of skin cancer, with over 200,000 new cases per year reported in the United States. The highest incidence occurs in Australia, where the age-adjusted incidence has been calculated to be 1332 cases per 100,000 population for men and 755 cases per 100,000 population for women. In European countries, the annual rate of incidence of SCC is about 25 cases per 100,000 people. SCC is an invasive tumour , which grows faster than BCC. SCC has a more aggressive behaviour, and his metastatic potential is about 2%-5%, like reported by Beauleau Lacoste et al. 1993, Postelthwaith et al. 1993 and Tavin et al. 1995; like BCC, SCC is often locally recurrent (Lee et al. 1985). Extension is often diffuse in the paths of cutaneous adnexae, and some times a perineural invasion is observed (Lawrence et al. 1994).It may appear everywhere on body skin surface, and may also come out on lips, vulva and penis. It often arises in some pre-existing cutaneous lesions, as chronic radiation keratosis, actinic keratosis, burn scars, hydrocarbon keratosis, arsenical keratosis and chronic skin ulcers. The early onset is an intraepidermal SCC (in situ), that also comprises morphologic forms as AK, Bowen's disease, and erythroplasia of Queyrat. Another particular form of SCC is   keratoacanthoma, characterized by a bulge or thick mass, often ulcerated; it evolves rapidly, and appears more frequently on exposed skin; the clinical invasive forms are the noduloulcerative and the verrucous one. AK and SCC frequently occur as multiple primary tumours in the same skin area ("field") in close proximity each other ("field cancerization") (Slaughter 1953), and its cells appear histologically similar to differentiated suprabasal keratinocytes. The risk factors include sun exposure (Gallagher et al. 1995), exposure to ionizing radiation (Lichter et al. 2000), arsenic exposure (Guo et al. 2001), coal tar derivates (Goldberg 1996), oral methoxsalen (psoralen) and ultraviolet-A radiation exposure (Nijsten et al. 2003). It is also recognized the importance of commonly predisponent factors, like immunosuppression (Jemec et al. 2003

1. The Diagnosis

Anamnesis and objective examination of the lesions by an experienced dermatologist is of fundamental importance for a correct diagnosis. Nevertheless, the current standard diagnostic procedure for NMSC is histologic examination, after excisional or incisional biopsy; sometimes a simple cytological examination of the scarified lesion is sufficient to confirm the diagnosis. In spite of this, there is increasing interest in non-invasive optical technologies for evaluation , diagnosis, and after-therapy monitoring, of skin cancer*in vivo*. Dermoscopy, or epiluminescence, is a very useful technique, of growing importance, for dermatological usage, and   represents a link between the clinical and the histological "viewpoints". It is largely employed for the diagnosis of pigmented lesions, and its use can strongly improve an early diagnosis of skin melanoma, but can also increases the diagnostic accuracy for many other skin pathologies, like BCC, AK, SCC, dermatofibroma, acanthoma, fibroepitelioma, angioma, inflammatory diseases. The dermoscopic characteristics features observed in BCC are   arborizing telangiectasia, blue/gray ovoid nests, ulceration, multiple blue/gray globules , leaf-like areas , and spoke-wheel areas (Altamura   2010). The dermoscopic features observed in SCC are less specific: multicomponent general pattern, whitish areas, scaly and crust elements, ulcerations, and hairpin vessels; in Bowen's disease a vascular pattern, mainly dotted and glomerular vessels, is a characteristic element. More recently, Reflectance Confocal Microscopy (RCM), an innovative optical technology for evaluation of normal and diseased skin in vivo, has been proposed for the diagnostics of BCC and the assessment of tumour margins prior to surgery (Sauermann et al. 2002). RCM of BCC lesions shows a nuclear pleomorphism at the level of the granular and spinous layer, superficial distruption and atypia of keratinocytes, nesting of atypical basal cells, increased blood vessel tortuosity, and nuclear polarization were typical markers for BCC (Astner et al. 2008).   Due to the high risk of recurrence of both BCC and SCC an accurate periodical examination of the patients is mandatory. Clinical exams include a full body skin examination, palpation of previous excision sites, examination of treated skin by dermoscopyand, if possible, by RCM. A check for possible metastasis is always mandatory; regional lymph nodes should be palpated for lymphadenopathy, and any suspicious lymph node enlargement should be evaluated by biopsy, imaging, or both. Imaging techniques using US, CT or CT/PET are useful for staging and detecting distant disease. MRI provides superior resolution of soft tissue tumours, particularly in the head and neck region, and should be considered for metastases that occur in these regions. Sentinel lymph node localisation and lymphoscintigraphy by ^{99m}Tc colloid should also be included, before and after therapy, on all suspect cases. Characteristics of primary tumours that develop into metastatic SCC include diameters >120mm^2, invasion to a depth >3.2 mm, and invasion of underlying fat, muscle or bone.

2. The Current Therapies

For both BCC and SCC tumours, standard therapies like curettage and electrodessication, surgery, cryosurgery (Margoob et al. 1997, Martinez et al. 2001), and intralesional interferon therapy (Cornell et al. 1992) are often proposed to the patients. In a long-term study (Fleming et al. 1995), BCC relapses have been observed, with tumour presence in the margins of histopathological smear in 39% of the cases after 5 years, and in 33% of the cases if the tumour was observed in the deep margin. New alternative topical therapy are now available for the treatment of selected cases, such as tumours located in critical, or inoperable patients, owing to systemic underlying diseases (cardiomyopathy, pulmonary insufficiency). They include imiquimod, an immune response modifier, approved for the treatment of superficial BCC less than 2 cm in diameter (Peris et al. 2005, Geisse et al. 2004); tazarotene, a retinoic acid, generally used for topical treatment of psoriasis, and proposed for the local treatment of BCC (Bianchi et al. 2004); photodynamic therapy, which involves the administration of a tumour-localizing photosensitizing agent and its subsequent activation with visible light to cause selective destruction of the tumour (Peng et al. 1997). The use of 5% imiquimod cream was an effective treatment option for superficial and nodular basal cell carcinomas, giving a clearance rate of 89.5% at an average of 39 months of follow up (Vun et al. 2006). The use of photodynamic therapy with porfimer sodium at 1 mg/kg produced, at 5-year, recurrence rates of 28%, and 15% for sporadic and nevoid basal cell carcinoma syndrome (NBCCS) lesions, respectively (Oseroff et al. 2006). By the use of meso-tetra-hydroxyphenyl-chlorin (mTHPC) mediated photodynamic therapy, good cosmetic results, with little or no scarring, were obtained in 87% of the treated lesions (Triesscheijn et al. 2006).

All these treatments are used for small, superficial and not recurrent BCC, but are not indicated for nodular, cystic, infiltrative and morphoeic variants. The current surgery practice is widespread performed, with margins of 2-4 mm recommended for nodular, well delineated, tumours sized up to 2 cm; for those larger than 2 cm, excision with margin of 1 cm, or more, is usually suggested, especially for tumours with aggressive course. Mohs' technique offers the best chances for cure and maximally preserves healthy tissue; it basically consists in the progressive histological real-time examination of tissue sections of the lesion during the surgery, up to the reaching of the healthy tissue (Petrovic et al. 2004). In all cases in which tumours are located in areas on which surgery excision may be very difficult (ear, nose, eyelids), the aesthetic and functional are often highly unsatisfactory (Garcia et al. 2006). When the lesion is rather large, and the residual healthy skin is not sufficient for a satisfactory surgical suture, it is necessary to proceed to a plastics reconstructive surgery, with transplantation of healthy skin (from the inferior limb, arm or gluteus skin). The cosmetic outcome is often unsatisfactory; if a relapse raise in transplanted skin, the management of the lesions becomes highly problematic.

Irradiation by photons has been used to deliver doses ranging from 20 to 73 Gy, in single or multiple treatments of BCC. The 5-year local control rate for recurrent Stage I and II carcinomas was 95%. These results suggested that high cure rates can be obtained in basal cell carcinomas treated with radiation therapy, with cure rates comparable to Mohs micrographic surgery (Wilder et al. 1991).

Squamous cell cancers have been treated with surgery followed by adjuvant radiation therapy, and irradiation confers a 5-year disease control probability of 0.79, while irradiation alone for untreated primary lesions, for recurrent primary lesions, or for untreated nodal metastases confers a disease control probability of approximately 0.50 (Shimm et al. 1991). Irradiation by conventional methods, due to the penetrating nature of the photons, cannot generally be recommended for treatment of tumours in areas in which radiation can be very harmful (face, eyes), and has proven itself often unsatisfactory in the treatment of SCC.

The interstitial brachtherapy with needles or seeds of ^{192}Ir been employed in cases of SCC of the penis (T1, T2 and T3, and also in the carcinoma in-situ). The results significantly change with tumour grade; the preservation of the penis after 5 years has been 86% of all treated cases.In a study from 1999 to 2004 (Skowronek et al), 179 patients with skin tumor (BCC and SCC) were treated with HDR brachytherapy, with 50 – 60 Gy in five or six fractions. Complete remission, 4 weeks after treatment, was observed in 84.9% of patients, partial remission in 8.9%, no remission in 9 5%.After 12 months, complete remission in 81.6% oft the cases, and progression in 8.9% were observed, respectively Higher remission rate is observed in tumors in lower clinical stage, treated radically and localised in the face. A group of patients were treated to varioussites, including lesions of the face and scalp, with Leipzig Surface Applicators to treat squamous or basal cell carcinomasabout2 cm in diameter (Musmacher et al). A custom surface mold applicator (FreiburgFlap) was used for lesions up to 4 cm; planning target volumeincluded the tumor plus a 5 mm margin. Treatment was delivered by HDR Brachytherapy(Ir-192), 5 Gy per fraction, twice per week for four weeks toa 5 mm depth. Results demonstrated the technique to be highly effective treatmentof skin carcinomas.

3. Brachytherapy Treatment by Beta Emitting Isotopes

In the present paper a beta emitter isotope brachytherapy therapeutic option for the treatment of BCC and of SCC is described. It basically consists in a superficial radiotherapy, characterized by the use of radioactive beta-emitting isotopes, incorporated in a specially formulated inert, synthetic matrix. The application product, based on a synthetic polymeric matrix containing a radioactive beta-emitting isotope, is easily applied on the surface of every BCC and SCC tumour, independently from its extension and lesion site. When the product is applied on the lesion, a beta emitter brachytherapy irradiation is performed, strictly limited to the area and depth affected by the tumour invasion. It can adapt itself to every skin surface, imparting an accurate distribution of dose and sparing the healthy tissue. The therapy has been used in a large variety of BCC and SCC forms, from tumours of very large sizes to relapsing or recurrent forms, to multifocal lesions (SEDDA et al 2003).

3.1. Materials and Methods

A ready-to-use, radioactive certified kit product (Re-SCT^{TM} , ITM,Munich, Germany) containing the ^{188}Re emitter has been used. The product is basically a mixture of ready-to-use synthetic resins and tensioactives, containing a certified dispersion of a ^{188}Re containing nanocolloid. The skin to be treated was protected with a thin layer of a hydrophobic/hydrophilic ointment (MAVIMED-Mavi, Italy) and with a specially designed, flexible thin plastic foil, in order to prevent any physical contact of the epidermiswith the radioactive matrix, and the kit product was applied above the protection layer. After some minutes the product solidified, without appreciable shrinkage; the radioactive mould was kept on the lesion for the time necessary to impart the calculated dose distribution. The product and the protection layer(s) thickness were accurately measured, in order to account for the beta radiation absorption effects. For each geometry, the dose distribution depends from the initial radioactivity, isotope emission energy, surface of the lesion and contact time.

3.2. Therapy Rationale of the Proposed Technique

The ^{188}Re isotope is a beta – gamma emitter; the ß-particleshave a maximal energy of 2.12 MeV and a mean energy of 764 keV, and the half-life of ^{188}Re is 16.98 hours.A γ-ray component of 155 keV accounts for 15% of theradiation intensity and allows excellent control of a possible contamination.The isotope ^{188}Re is easily available as certified isotope, and the high-energy ß particles of ^{188}Re are therapeutically effective only at short ranges, sparing the health tissue from unwanted irradiation, which is the typical drawback of X-ray and gamma radiotherapy treatments.The dose distribution of beta particles in human tissue is well described by a complex exponential function of the form

$$D(x)=K \ (c(1\text{-}vx \ e \ 1\text{-}(vx/c))+vx \ e \ 1\text{-}(vx/c))$$

$$(vx)2 \ c$$

where $(1\text{-}vx \ e^{\ 1\text{-}(vx/c)}) = 0$ for $x >$ c/v, D(x) is the dose rate at distance x from the source, v is the absorption coefficient, k is a normalization constant, c is a dimensionless parameter.

Due to the penetrating nature of X-ray and gamma photons, as in classical radiotherapy, an irradiation of skin tumours often requires many sessions, and imparts a non-negligible dose to underlying tissue, so arising the possibility of long term after effects. The electrons from high energy (> 1MeV) beta emitters isotopes deposit more than 90 % of the dose to the first two mm of the skin, which is the depth usually interested from tumour invasion, but spare the irradiation of deeper tissue. Typical real case dose absorption curves in human tissue for the beta emitter ^{188}Re are reported in the Figure 1.

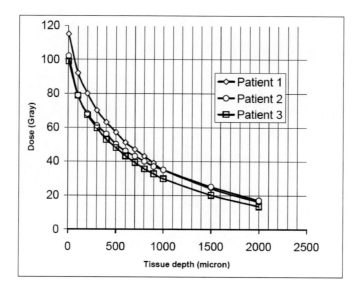

Figure 1. Typical dose deposition curve of the beta emitter resin on the skin of the patients.

4. Patient Preparation before the Treatment

The application of the product must be preceded by an accurate cleaning and curettage of the lesions. This treatment is useful not only for more precisely delineate the borders of a tumour, but also to eliminate all the hyperkeratosis , granulation tissue, scabs, that, due to their thickness, would stop the beta particles irradiation.Both BCC and SCC appear often ulcerated, with presence of serous and blood scabs, in other cases keratin plaques or nodules of horny consistence are present; in all cases an accurate and complete preliminary elimination of this material must be performed. A softening of the scab with saline helps in the removing; in some cases, like vulva or penis lesions, a local anaesthesia before removing is advisable. If, after the removal of the scab, a haemorrhage arises, an haemostatic agent must be applied on the lesion, to completely stop the bleeding.

The area to be treated is outlined by using accurate visual examination and epiluminescence; the irradiation usually includes both the area of evident infiltration, and the area in which a neoangiogenic development is present; a border of some mm of apparently health tissue around the lesion is also usually included in the irradiation area, especially if a possible invasion is suspected, particularly in the "field cancerization" cases.

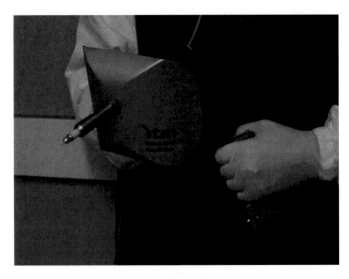

Figure 2. Shielded device for the application of the radioactive beta emitter resin on the tumour lesion.

5. Application of the Product

The clinical practice has showed that the inclusion of a border of two-five mm (depending from the size of the lesion) beyond the visible invasion and neoangiogenic development, is sufficient to assure a selective irradiation in most cases. The surface to be treated is outlined by a dermographic pen, and the drawing is transferred on a transparent thin plastic sheet settled on the lesion, from which a determination of the area is performed by an image analyzer. The whole surface of the skin to be treated is protected by uniformly spreading it with a calculated layer of a special gel cream an/or of a specially designed inert plastic thin foil. The gel rapidly desiccates, leaving an adhering, uniform and continuous protection film, with typical final thickness of 30-40 microns.The radioactive product Re-SCT^{TM} has a uniformly distributed and certified radioactivity, and must be applied as accurately and homogeneously as possible, by covering all the previously outlined area. The application of the product on the skin was performed by the use of a shielded dedicated applicator (Figure 2). A Perspex screen 10 mm thick is sufficient to protect the physician face from β radiation during the phase of product application to the patient, typically lasting from 30 to 120 seconds. During the irradiation, typically lasting from 15 min to 1 hour, the patient is kept isolated. If an irradiation on the nose or near the eye is performed, the patient wears a pair of lead or *polymethylmethacrylate* spectacles, for crystalline protection. The dose to the hands of medical personnel during the application was found within acceptable levels (< 2 mSv).

The radioactive mould is kept on the lesion for the time necessary to impart the calculated dose distribution. For each lesion, the dose distribution only depends from the initial radioactivity, surface of the lesion and contact time. For each patient and for each lesion, the dose-distribution curve is calculated by using a point source real-time integration software program. Clinical practice has demonstrated that mean doses of 40–60 Gy to depths of 300–600 microns from the epidermis (the exact value depending on histological indications and site of the tumour) are effective for high cure rates. A dose of 50 Gy to 300 microns has been used in lesion of genitals, lips and mouth; 50 Gy to 400 or 500 microns was the standard dose used for most of the BCC and SCC lesions, 50 Gy to 600 microns was the dose used in thick tumours.At the end of the irradiation, the resin was removed, by using a specially designed shielded tongs device.

6. Typical Clinical Results after the Treatment

Immediately after the treatment a faint reddening of the treated areawas visible. After a few days a variable erythema was present, sometimes with emission of serum, and a crust or scab was formed. An apparent worsening of the aspect of the lesion was often observed, with the appearance of a light burn, but the bleeding, often present before the therapy, usually disappeared. After 40-120 days the erythema faded, sometimes a second scab formed, and itch was sometimes present; the clinical healing was more clearly apparent, the tumour neoangiogenic development, often clearly visible with epiluminescence before the treatment, started to disappear. After 60-180 days, in most of the cases, an apparent clinical healing was noted, rarely with persistence of a scab (SEDDA et al. 2007); the lesion area became paler than the untreated skin, and the tumour neoangiogenic development disappeared.More than 350 patients (for a total of almost 1200 lesions) with histologically or clinically confirmed diagnosis of BCC and of SCC have been up today successfully treated. In most of the treated cases, an apparent clinical remission occurred after 3-9 months. After a follow up of 12 - 78 months a complete response was obtained in 98.5% of all the treated lesions, in 89 % of the lesions after a single application. In such cases, when a histological examination was performed, a complete tumour regression was observed. In 11% of the patients, two to three treatments were applied. In half of these cases the second treatment was applied on lesions contiguous to the treated area, or to the border of the previously treated lesions; in such cases the evaluation of the area interested from the tumour invasion has been likely underestimated. In some cases, thicker tumours generally required two or even three treatments (i.e. keratoacanthoma, or thick nodular BCC), as was easily foreseen by purely dosimetric consideration. In a limited number of cases multiple treatments (maximum three) on the same area have been found necessary for a complete healing; possible reasons should be a greater radio-resistance of the tumour cell line, or a protective effect of the melanin (pigmented BCC). Neither un-aesthetic scars, nor side effects, were generally observed. The 1.5% of the cases in which a complete healing has not been reached, were mainly old, inoperable patients in which a deep tissue invasion was present, and have been enrolled only as compassionate cases. Some examples of obtained clinical results are reported from Figure 3 to Figure 13.

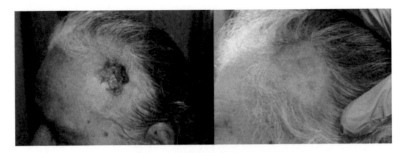

Figure 3. Ulcerated BCC of the scalp, and 382 days after a single treatment.

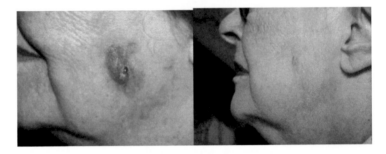

Figure 4. SCC of the face before, and 181 days after a single treatment.

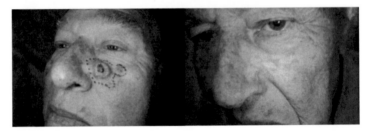

Figure 5. Keratoacanthoma before the treatment, and 180 days after two treatments.

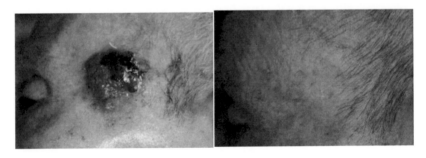

Figure 6. Wide ulcerated SCC of the temple before, and 83 days after a single treatment.

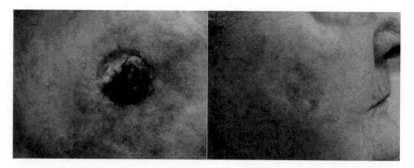

Figure 7. SCC of the face before, and 134 days after a single treatment.

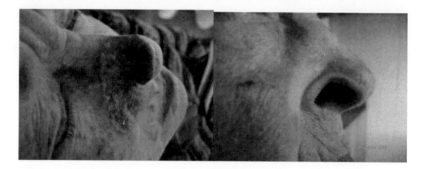

Figure 8. Ulcerated BCC of the nose, extended to the face, before, and 151 days after a single treatment.

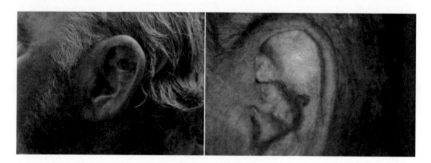

Figure 9. SCC of the ear before, and 455 days after two treatment.

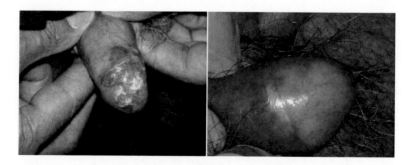

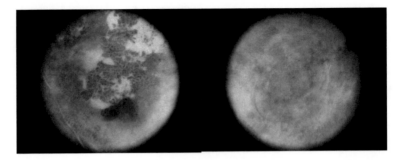

Figure 10. SCC of the penis before, and 405 days after two treatments.

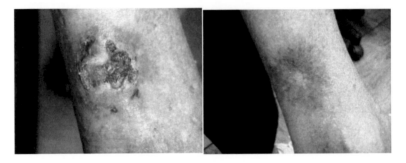

Figure 11. Ulcerated SCC of the leg before, and 483 days after a single treatment; picture and dermoscopy of the lesion.

7. Conclusions

The results obtained by using the described product forbeta emitter brachytherapycan be considered quite satisfactory for the great majority of treated patients, and is proposed as a herapeutic choice, not only alternative to medical treatments, but also to surgery.Modern fractionated dose radiotherapy is an extremely useful form of treatment, and can be used to treat many forms of cancer, but often faces the same problem of accurately identifying tumour margins as standard excision surgery, due to the lack of individually moulded radiation collimators. The treatment of tumours in areas in which radiation can be very harmful is some times problematic, due to the penetrating nature of gamma photons or X rays.In this respect the use of the beta radiation embedded in a taylor-made irradiation mould, like the technique described in the present paper, can override the drawbacks of classical radiotherapy. It must be noted that the mean dose distribution curves corresponding to performed treatments (Figure 1) shows a clear falloff in dose from a nominal value of 100 - 120 Gy in the epidermis, to less than 20 Gy at a depth of only 2 mm, a value sometimes considered interested from invasion in this class of tumours. Single fraction radiotherapy has been used for the treatment of small superficial BCC and SCC in more than 800 patients, obtaining an overall disease-free rate at 5 years of 84%; the optimal applied dose for such a lesion on a flat surface was 20 Gy (CHAN et al. 2007). So, the dose distribution curve obtained by beta particles irradiation apparently seems to ideally "follow" the distribution of the tumour invasion in the dermal tissue, administering the therapeutic dose only at the required depth, without unnecessary dose deposition in the subdermal tissue. The choice of the apparently healthy tissue to be included in the irradiation is an important parameter, because a lethal dose must be administered to the potentially infiltrating cells in the external border. A complete histological examination for the whole lesion area is seldom present, due to its invasiveness, and the dermatologist examination and the doctor personal experience is of utmost importance in the choice of the irradiation limit.After the dermatological examination, the application of a taylor-made radioactive product over the lesion offers the possibility to perform a conformational radiotherapy, using the real tumour border, independently from the shape complexity and number of the lesions.

It has also recently been recognized that doses of radiation, lower than or equal to those that cause direct cytolysis, may alter the phenotype of target tissue by up-regulating gene products that may make tumour cells more susceptible to T-cell-mediated immune attack (GARNETT et al. 2004). So, it cannot be excluded a synergistic mechanism in the clinical and histological healing of tumour lesions apparently thicker than the beta particles therapeutic range.

Apart from the underlying mechanism, the main advantage of the described technique lies in the usefulness in all types of BCC and SCC, without restriction of site, dimension, clinical or histological type, and patient clinical situation. A superiority of the proposed treatment respect to the surgery is evident for all the tumours located in high-risk areas, or difficult sites on which surgery would be difficult (nose, ears, eyelids), in the patients with a high number of lesions or with tumour relapses, in patients in which surgery would produce functional mutilations (penis, vulva, eyelids lesions), and, generally, in older, infirm, or otherwise inoperable patients (SEDDA et al. 2008).Avoidance of scarring and of suboptimal cosmetic outcome were also considered by patients an important decision factor in the choice of this therapeutic path. The proposed technique is a rapid, safe, treatment, mostly performed in a single therapeutic session, without discomfort for the patient, and offers a complete aesthetical and functional *restitutio ad integrum*.

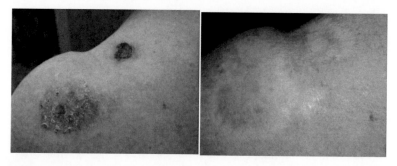

Figure 12. Multifocal BCC of the shoulder before, and 154 days after a single treatment.

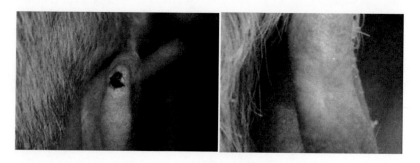

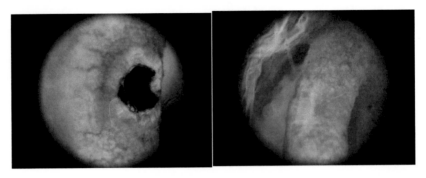

Figure 13. BCC of the ear leg before, and 154 days after a single treatment; picture and dermoscopy of the lesion.

References

Altamura, D; Menzies, SW; Argenziano, G; Zalaudek, I; Soyer, HP; Sera, F; Avramidis, M; DeAmbrosis, K; Fargnoli, MC; Peris, K. Dermatoscopy of basal cell carcinoma: morphologic variability of global and local features and accuracy of diagnosis, *JAmAcadDermatol*, 2010, 62(1), 67-75. Epub 2009 Oct 13.

American Cancer Society. Cancer Facts and Figures. ACS: Atlanta. http://www.cancer

Armstrong, B; Kricker, A. The epidemiology of UV induced skin cancer, *JPhotochemPhotobiol*, 2001, B63, 8-18.

Astner, S; Dietterle, S; Otberg, N; Röwert-Huber, HJ; Stockfleth, E; Lademann, J. Clinical applicability of in vivo fluorescence confocal microscopy for noninvasive diagnosis and therapeutic monitoring of nonmelanoma skin cancer, *JBiomedOpt.*, 2008 Jan-Feb, 13(1).

Beauleu Lacoste, I; Joly, P; Ruto, F; Thomine, F; Fusade, T; Chevaillier, B; Ortoli, JC; Lauret, P. Metastatic basal cell carcinoma, *Ann-Dermatol-Venerol*, 1993, 120(2), 135-138.

Bianchi, L; Orlandi, A; Campione, E. Topical treatment of basal cell carcinoma with tazarotene: a clinicopathological study on a large series of cases, *Br J Dermatol*, 2004, 151, 148-56.

Bowden, G; Prevention of non-melanoma skin cancer by targeting ultraviolet-B-light signalling, *NatRevCancer*, 2004, 4, 23-35.

Cassarino, DS; Derienzo, PD; Barr, RJ. Cutaneous squamous cell carcinoma: a comprehensive clinicopathologic classification-Part II, *J Cutan Pathol*, 2006, Apr, 33(4), 261-79.

Chan, S;Dhadda, AS;Swindell, R. Single fraction radiotherapy for small superficial carcinoma of the skin, *ClinOncol*, (R Coll Radiol), 2007 May, 19(4), 256-9.

Cornell, RC; Greenway, HT; Tucker, S; Edwards, L; Ashworth, S; Vance, J; Tanner, D. Intralesional interferon therapy for basal cell carcinoma. J.Am.Acad. *Dermatology*, 1990, 23 (4), 694-700.

Diepgen, T; Mahler, V. The epidemiology of skin cancer, *Br J Dermatol*, 2002, 146 (Suppl 61), 1-6.

Fleming, I; Amonette, MD; Managhan, T; Fleming, I. Principles of Management of basal and squamous cell carcinoma of the skin, *Cancer*, 1995, 75 (suppl. No 2), 699-704.

Fu, W; Cockerell, C. The actinic keratosis: a 21st-century perspective, *ArchDermatol*, 2003, 139, 66-70.

Gallagher, RP; Hill, GB; Bajdik, CD; et All. Sunlight exposure, pigmentary factors, and risk of non melanocytic skin cancer. I. Basal cell carcinoma, *ArchDermatol*, 1995, 131, 157-63.

Garcia, L;Nagore, E;Llombart, B;Sanmartin, O;Botella-Estrada, R;Requena, C;Jorda, E;Guillen, C.Basal cell carcinoma of the nasolabial fold: an apparently 'benign' tumour that often needs complex surgery,*J Eur Acad Dermatol Venereol*, 2006 Sep, 20(8), 926-30.

Garnett, CT;Palena, C;Chakraborty, M;Tsang, KY;Schlom, J;Hodge, JW. Sublethal irradiation of human tumor cells modulates phenotype resulting in enhanced killing by cytotoxic T lymphocytes, *Cancer Res.*, 2004 Nov, 1, 64(21), 7985-94.

Geisse, J; Caro, I. Lindholm J Imiquimod 5% cream for the treatment of superficial basal cell carcinoma: results from two phase III, randomized, vehicle controlled studies, *JAmAcadDermatol*, 2004, 50, 722-33.

Goldberg, LH. Basal cell carcinoma, *Lancet*, 1996, 347, 663-667.

Guo, HR; Yu, HS; Hu, H; Monson, RR. Arsenic in drinking water and skin cancers: Cell type specificity (Taiwan, ROC). *CancerCausesControl*, 2001, 12, 909-16.

Jemec, JB; Holm, EA. Non-melanoma skin cancer in organ transplant patients, *Transplantation*, 2003, 75, 253-7.

Jih, D; Lyle, S; Elenitsas, R; Elder, D; Cotsarelis, G. Cytokeratin 15 expression in trichoepiteliomas and a subset of basal cell carcinomas suggests they originate from hair follicle stem cells, *J Cutan Pathol*, 1999, 26, 113-118.

Lawrence N; Cottel WI: Squamous cell carcinoma of skin with perineural invasion, *JAmAcadDermatol*, 1994 Jul, 31(1), 30-3

Lee, K; McKean, ME; McGregor, IA. Metastatic patterns of squamous carcinoma in the parotid lymph nodes, *BrJPlastSurg.*, 1985 Jan, 38(1), 6-10.

Lichter, MD; Karagas, MR; Mott, LA; Spencer, SK; et All. Therapeutic ionizing Radiation and the incidence of basal cell carcinoma and squamous cell carcinoma, *ArchDermatol*, 2000, 136, 1007-11.

Margoob, AA. Basal and squamous cell carcinomas: what every primary care physician should know, *PostgradMed*, 1997, 102, 139-59.

Marks, R; Rennie, G; Selwood, T. Malignant transformation of solar keratosis to squamous cell carcinoma, *Lancet*, 1988, 1, 795-797.

Martinez, JC; Otley, CC. The management of melanoma and non-melanoma skincancer: a review for the primary care physician, *MayoClinicProc.*, 2001, 76, 1253 63.

Musmacher, J; Ghaly, M; Satchwill, K.High dose rate brachytherapy with surface applicators: Treatment for nonmelanomatous skin cancer,*JournalofClinicalOncology*, ASCO Annual Meeting Proceedings (Post-Meeting Edition), 2006 24 (18s) (June 20 Supplement), 15543.

Nijsten, TE; Stern, RS. The increased risk of skin cancer is persistent after discontinuation of psoralen+ultraviolet A: a cohort study, *J Invest Dermatol*, 2003, 121, 252-8.

Nindl, I; Gottschling, M; Stockfleth, E. Human Papillomaviruses and non-melanoma skin cancer: Basic virology and clinical manifestations, *Disease Markers*, 2007, 23, 247-259.

Oseroff, AR;Blumenson, LR;Wilson, BD;Mang, TS;Bellnier, DA;Parsons, JC;Frawley, N;Cooper, M;Zeitouni, N;Dougherty, TJ. A dose ranging study of photodynamic therapy with porfimer sodium (Photofrin) for treatment of basal cell carcinoma,*Lasers Surg Med*, 2006 Jun, 38(5), 417-26.

Peng, Q; Warloe, T; Ber,g. K; Moan, J; Kongshaug, M; Gierksky, KE; Nesland, JM. 5-Aminolevulinic acid-based photodynamic theraphy: clinical research and future challenges, *Cancer*, 1997, 79, 2282-308.

Peris, K; Campione, E. Micantonio T Imiquimod treatment of superficial and nodular basal cell carcinoma: 12 week open label trial, *DermatolSurg*, 2005, 31, 318-23.

Petrovic, D; Visnjic, M; Mihailovich, D; Petrovic, S; Pesic, Z. Margin size in basocellular skin carcinoma resection: impact on relapse, *Acta Fac Med Naiss*, 2004, 21(4), 195-200.

Postelthwaith, KR; Courteney, DJ; Gosney, JR. Basal cell carcinoma with hepatic metastases, *J Oral Maxillofac Surg.*, 1993, 50, 670-673.

Roewert-Huber, J; Lange-Asschenfeldt, B; Stockfleth, E and Kerl H; Epidemiology and aetiology of basal cell carcinoma, *Br J Dermatol*, 2007, 157(S2), 47-51.

Sauermann, K; Gambichler, T; Wilmert, M; Rotterdam, S; Stücker, M; Altmeyer, P; Hoffmann, K. Investigation of basal cell carcionoma by confocal laser scanning microscopy in vivo, *Skin Research and Technology,8(3)*, 141-147.

Sedda, AF; Rossi, G; Cipriani, C. Beta emitter multilayer for the dermatological brachytherapy of cutaneous tumours, European Association of Nuclear Medicine- *Annual Congress*, Amsterdam, September 2003.

Sedda, AF; Rossi, G; Cipriani, C; Carrozzo, AM; Donati, P. Dermatological beta brachytherapy of basal and squamous cell carcinoma, *21st World Congress of Dermatology*, 30 September-5 October 2007 Buenos Aires .

Sedda, AF; Rossi, G; Cipriani, C; Carrozzo, AM; Donati, P. Dermatological high-dose-rate brachytherapy for the treatment of basal and squamous cell carcinoma, *Clinical and Experimental Dermatology*, Volume 33 Issue 6, Pages 745-749 (November 2008)

Shimm, DS; Wilder, RB. Radiation therapy for squamous cell carcinoma of the skin, *Am J Clin Oncol*, 1991, 14, 383-386.

Skowronek, J; Chicheł, A; Piotrowski, T. HDR brachytherapy of skin cancer – the Wielkopolski Cancer Centre's experience, *Współcz Onkol*, 2005,9(8), 347-354.

Slaughter, D; Southwick, H; Smejkal, W. Field cancerization in oral stratified squamous epithelium; clinical implications of multicentric origin, *Cancer*, 1953, 6, 963-968.

Tavin, E; Persy, MS; Jacobs, J. Metastatic basal cell carcinoma of the head and neck, *Laryngoscope*, 1995, 105 (8PH1), 814-817.

Triesscheijn, M;Ruevekamp, M;Antonini, N;Neering, H;Stewart, FA;Baas, P. Optimizing Meso-tetra-hydroxyphenyl-chlorin Mediated Photodynamic Therapy for Basal Cell Carcinoma, *Photochem Photobiol*,2006, 82(6), 1686-1690.

Vun, Y;Siller, G. Use of 5% imiquimod cream in the treatment of facial basal cell carcinoma: a 3-year retrospective follow-up study, *Australas J Dermatol*, 2006 Aug, 47(3), 169-71.

Wilder, RB; Kittelson, JM; Shimm, DS. Basal Cell Carcinoma treated with radiation therapy, *Cancer*, 1991, 68, 2134-37.

In: Brachytherapy
Editor: Leoni M. Fische

ISBN: 978-1-61728-750-3
© 2011 Nova Science Publishers, Inc.

Chapter 5

Intracavitary Accelerated Partial Breast Irradiation

Daniel J. Scanderbeg and
Catheryn M. Yashar
Department of Radiation Oncology
University of California, San Diego, California, USA

1.1 Introduction

Breast cancer treatment has changed substantially in the past several decades. Initially, all women were treatment with mastectomy. However, this is a major and often a very difficult surgery for the patient, both physically and emotionally. Several studies were published that demonstrated acceptable local control and equivalent survival when mastectomy was compared with whole breast irradiation (WBI) following the surgical removal of the tumor[1,2].This shifted the treatment paradigm as the new standard of care became 5 – 6 weeks of radiation delivered to the whole breast. Although a survival benefit for WBI has not been demonstrated in prospective, randomized trials, a metaanalysis suggests that there may be a small benefit for women less than 60 years of age [3].

There has been a recent attempt to shift the treatment paradigm, once again, in order to minimize the amount of normal tissueexposed to radiationand also shorten the overall treatment time. This new treatment, accelerated partial breast irradiation (APBI), is completed in 5 days.APBI includes resection of the tumor followed by focused radiation to the tissue adjacent to the tumorbed where historical data demonstrates is the most likely area of breast cancer recurrence [4]. Additionally, multicentric disease at presentation, while possible, is not common. Tumor recurrences far from the index lesion are often molecularly distinct from the index lesions and have not been shown to be preventable with whole breast irradiation indicating the benefit of WBI is to eliminate cancer cells inadvertently left behind at the time of surgery [5]. Accelerated partial breast irradiation can be delivered with external beam radiotherapy or high-dose-rate (HDR) brachytherapy. High-dose-rate brachytherapy can be delivered via interstitial needles or an intracavitary device. With any of the modalities, the target dose is delivered on an outpatient basis, twice daily,over 5 days [6-8]. Hence, it is much faster than conventional radiotherapy (5-6 weeks) and is convenient for women who desire or need treatment on an accelerated schedule for numerous reasons, such as work schedule, living far from the treatment center, etc.

There have been several studies that have demonstrated equivalent control between APBI and WBI, and there has been one randomized, prospective trial that has demonstratedequal local control at 5 years, and better cosmesis in the APBI arm[9-11]. Currently, the National Cancer Institute (NCI), the National Surgical Adjuvant Breast and Bowel Project (NSABP-39), and the Radiation Therapy Oncology Group (0413) are sponsoring a prospective, randomized trial in North America.Upon registration, patients are randomizedto WBI orAPBI using one of three methods:interstitial brachytherapy, 3D conformal radiotherapy, or MammoSite® RTS(Hologic, Inc., Bedford, MA)balloon brachytherapy. There are numerous other trials attempting to answer this question of equivalence between WBI and APBI including the Canadian Ontario Clinical Oncology Group RAPID trial with 3Dconformal therapy, the Italian ELIOT study of intraoperative electrons, the Clinical Trials Group of the University College London TARGIT trial of targeted intraoperative radiotherapy, GEC-ESTRO (Groupe Européen de Curiethérapie - European Society for Therapeutic Radiology and Oncology) trial using interstitial brachytherapy, and the United Kingdom IMPORT LOW trial using intensity modulated radiation therapy for APBI. However, despite the paucity of randomized prospective data comparing APBI to WBI, the popularity of APBI is increasing rapidly. Due to this increase in popularity, several national groups, including the American Brachytherapy Society (ABS), the American Society of Breast Surgeons (ASBS), and the American Society for Therapeutic Radiology and Oncology (ASTRO) have all published guidelines on the use of APBI outside of a protocol setting (Table 1) [12,13].

1.2 Treatment Modalities

There are numerous methods for breast irradiation, and each has its own history and published data set. In all, there is a large and rapidly changing body of work although this chapter will limit its review to intracavitary devices for APBI. However, it is important to be aware of the other techniques being employed at this time including interstitial brachytherapy, external beam 3D conformal and intensity modulated therapy, intraoperative therapy, and permanent seed implantation. The following sections include a brief introduction to these APBI techniques followed by an in-depth discussion of each of the intracavitary applicators.

1.2.1. Multi-Catheter Interstitial

Multi-catheterinterstitial brachytherapy was the initial method of APBI described, and still maintains the largest body of literature. It was initially used as a boost following whole breast irradiation. On average, 20 needles are placed through the tissue surrounding the lumpectomy site. Following catheter insertion and planning, radiation is delivered with a high-dose-rate afterloader. Patients are generally treated on an outpatient basis with twice daily radiation treatments, separated by a minimum of 6 hours. Data from the Oschner clinic phase I/II study showed similar outcomes with regards to local recurrence, grade III toxicity, and cosmesis scores when compared to external beam radiation therapy, with a median follow-up of 75 months[9].

Table 1. Patient selection criteria for APBI

	ABS	ASBS	ASTRO strict	ASTRO "with caution"	ASTRO on trial
Age	≥ 45	≥ 50	≥ 60	50-59	< 50
Diagnosis	Unifocal, invasive ductal carcinoma	Invasive ductal carcinoma or DCIS	Invasive ductal, mucinous, tubular, or colloid, no EIC or LVI, ER(+)	Invasive lobular, EIC < 3 cm, limited or focal LVI, ER(-), DCIS < 3 cm	Extensive LVI, pure DCIS > 3 cm, neoadjuvant chemo
Tumor Size	≤ 3 cm	≤ 3 cm	cUnifocal < 2 cm	2.1 – 3.0 cm	> 3 cm, T3, T4 or cmultifocal, multicentric
Surgical Margins	Negative microscopic surgical margins	Negative microscopic surgical margins of at least 2 mm	≥ 2 mm	< 2 mm	(+)
Nodal Status	N0	N0	N0 or IHC(+) only		N(+) or undissected

Another randomized study comparing WBI to interstitial brachytherapy by Polgar et al., with 5 year results, demonstrated similar local control and overall survival and also improved cosmesis in the interstitial arm [11]. Due to the numerous catheters placed around the target area, the radiation source has a large number of possible dwell positions allowing for the most conformance of dose to the target area; but,outcome depends on experience and expertisewith this technique. Interstitial breast brachytherapy is not commonly taught in North American radiation oncology residencies and is, therefore, not widely available in the United States. However, it is the most commonly accepted form of partial breast irradiation in Europe. One potential disadvantage to this technique is that numerous catheters may leave visible scars on the breast, especially noticeable with upper, inner quadrant lesions.

1.2.2 3dcrt

Three-dimensional conformal radiation therapy (3DCRT) is a less invasive, alternative form of APBI, which does not require a surgical procedure for applicator implantation, a distinct advantage of this treatment modality. In addition, while all radiation oncology practices have a linear accelerator, access to a HDR applicator is more limited. Using the accelerator external radiation beamsare focused on the target tissue adjacent to the lumpectomy cavity. The prescribed dose with this technique is typically 38.5 Gy over the course of 5 days, with treatments twice per day. Usually a 3 to 5 non-coplanar beam arrangement is used for treatment with none of the beams pointed at the heart, lung, or contralateral breast [14]. There is ongoing debate with this technique regarding the appropriate cavity margin to irradiate when respiratory motion and target placement uncertainty in a mobile breast are taken into account. However, due to these issues the margin around the tumor bed is necessarily increased compared to brachytherapy techniques. Using the necessary margin increases the amount of normal tissue exposed to irradiation. Also, due to the nature of external beam radiation (with a radiation entry and exit point), this method always delivers dose to more normal tissue than the other methods. Therefore, great care must be taken to plan avoid exit dose through normal, sensitive tissues such as heart, lung, shoulder, and contralateral breast. Excellent local control and cosmetic outcomehas been reported by Vicini et al. with minimal chronic toxicity at 2 years [15]. However,this method of delivery may be more toxic to normal tissue due to the higher dose per treatment used and unexpected toxicities have been reported [16,17]. Intensity modulated radiation therapy has also been used to increase the dose homogeneity and decrease normal tissue radiation exposure. Results from a randomized, prospective phase III trial are currently in press and the results, albeit with short follow-up, are promising [18].

1.2.3. Intra-Op Electrons

Another technique under active investigation is intra-operative electron radiotherapy (IORT). Immediately following tumor removal, a linear accelerator (positioned in the operating room) is used to deliver electron beam radiotherapy to the surgical field. All surrounding normal tissues such as the heart, thoracic wall, and lung are shielded. Promising IORT results were first reported by The University of Milan in 2001 and, since then, there have been published follow-up reportswith excellent treatment efficacy and minimal toxicity at 2 years [19]. Equivalent treatment efficacy and mild to moderate late toxicity has been reported by Mussari et al. with 4-year outcome data[20]. The main drawback with this technique is that many centers do not have the necessary equipment to perform this procedure.

1.2.4. Permanent Low-Dose-Rate Seed Implants

Much like permanent low-dose-rate prostate seed implants, the use of permanent seeds in the breast has also been investigated. Palladium (^{103}Pd) sources, with dimensions approximating a grain of rice, are implanted into the target tissue following lumpectomy. Zero local recurrence and minimal toxicity, at 32 months, has been recently reported by Pignol et al.from the outcome of a phase I/II study[21]. Questions regarding radiation exposure from this technique have been addressed and demonstrated safety for the public [22].

1.2.5. Intracavitary Devices

As of this writing, there are three intracavitary devices out on the market: Hologic, Inc.'s (Bedford, MA) MammoSite®, SenoRx's (Aliso Viejo, CA) Contura®, and Cianna Medical, Inc.'s (Aliso Viejo, CA) SAVI™, and each are described below. MammoSite® was the first intracavitary applicator on the market, followed by SAVI and Contura. Both the Contura and SAVI have multiple peripheral catheters that allow for shaping of dose and thereby more sparing of normal tissue, since the dose distribution can be non-spherical. In response to these devices, MammoSitehas recently released a redesigned multi-catheter balloon applicator; although the original single catheter applicator is still available for use.

1.2.5.1. Mammosite

MammoSite was the first single-entry balloon brachytherapy device used for APBI[23-29]. It gained FDA clearance in 2002 and since then has treated over 50,000 patients and greatly increased the popularity of APBI due to its ease of use. The MammoSiteapplicator has a double-lumen catheter with a silicone balloon at the distal tip and is shown in Figure 1. The double-lumen catheter has one port for balloon inflation and the other to house the radiation source, with both ports using a Luer Lock connection. The MammoSite balloon comes in two sizes (4-5 cm and 5-6 cm) in spherical balloon geometry, and a 4-6 cm elliptical balloon.

Surgical insertion can either be performed intra-operatively or post-operatively. In either case, after insertion of the device, the balloon is filled with a saline-contrast mixture so that it is visible using image modalities such as orthogonal x-rays or computed tomography (CT) (Figure 2).

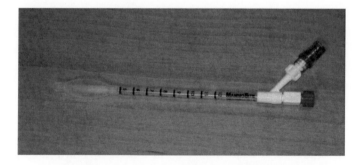

Figure 1.

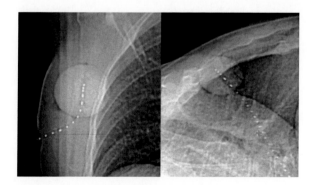

Figure 2.

With the MammoSite, dose is prescribed to a volume of tissueextending 1.0 cm from the balloon surface. This is in contrast to traditional interstitial brachytherapy that typically treats a margin around the lumpectomy cavity defined as a 1.5-2.0 cm expansion beyond the cavity wall. However, Dicker et al. published a study indicating that treating a 1.0 cm margin from the balloon surface effectively treats a mean tissue margin of 1.6 cm from the center of an empty lumpectomy cavity [30]. A subsequent study conducted by Edmundson et al. predicts a treatment margin of up to 2.0 cm [31]. Both reported that balloon expansion causes tissue stretching and when evaluated after balloon removal, an unstretched volume equivalent to 1.5-2 cm is effectively treated.

Table 2. Dosimetric guidelines for APBI techniques

	Interstitial	MammoSite	SAVI	Contura
V90	> 90%	> 90%	> 90%	>90%
V95	NA	NA	> 95%	>95%
V150	≤ 70 cc	≤ 50 cc	≤ 50 cc	≤ 50 cc
V200	≤ 20 cc	≤ 10 cc	≤ 20 cc	≤ 10 cc
Skin Dose	NA	≤ 145%	≤ 100%	≤ 125%

The radioactive source can be loaded in a linear configuration down the central catheter in the single catheter device and also linearly in the 3 peripheral catheters for the multi-lumen device. The dose distribution is approximately spherical for the single catheter device. Initially, due to the single catheter design and the symmetric, spherical dose distribution, the dose could not be adjusted to patient anatomy and hence reports began to emerge with safety guidelines that recommended the tissue bridge between the outside surface of the balloon and the patient's skin should not be less than 5 mm, and caution should be exercised when placed directly on the chest wall [32]. Published dosimetric constraints for this device, as well as the other intracavitary devices and interstitial, are shown in Table 2. These guidelines suggest that 90% of the target volume (PTV_eval) should receive at least 90% of the dose (V90% > 90%) and that the volume of target tissue receiving 150% (V150) and 200% (V200) of the dose should remain less than 50 cc and 10 cc, respectively. Additional constraints include a recommended skin bridge of at least 7 mm, but a minimum skin bridge of 5 mm, with a constraint on the skin dose, which must receive less than 145% of the prescribed dose.

With the single channel device, any rotation of the balloon will not affect the dose distribution. Therefore, daily quality assurance only needs to verify the balloon integrity and can be performed with orthogonal x-rays, a CT scan, or ultrasound.

To allow dose modulation for normal tissue sparing, Hologic, Inc. released a newly designed balloon applicator in late 2009 that has 4 catheters inside the balloon; one central catheter and 3 peripheral catheters, as well as changing the balloon material from silicone to polyurethane. These additional catheters help achieve better dosimetric conformity to the patient's anatomy by allowing dose shaping.

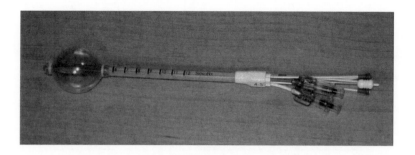

Figure 3.

Keisch et al. were the first to report on the MammoSite, demonstrating mild to moderate side-effects with its use[28]. Four year data from the American Society of Breast Surgeons registry reports treatment efficacy, toxicity, and cosmesis outcomes similar to comparable APBI techniques [29]. Benitez et al. reported on its use with excellent local control and minimal toxicity at 5-years, with some limitations caused by poor cavity conformance and inadequate skin distance in select patients[23].

1.2.5.2 Contura

SenoRx's Contura (Figure 3), is a multi-lumen balloon brachytherapy devicethat was the first to combine a balloon applicator with multi-catheter technology and gained FDA clearance in 2007. The balloon is a spherical shape and made from polyurethane. The Contura comes in 2 different sizes (a 4-5 cm balloon and a 5-6 cm balloon) depending on the volume of the lumpectomy cavity Table 3, same as the MammoSite. The Contura has 5 catheters, with all the catheters contained inside the balloon. There are two Luer lock connectors at the proximal end, one for inflation of the balloon and one for vacuum suction. The vacuum port runs along the end of the catheter to the tip and allows for suction to be applied to remove seroma or air that remains outside the balloon to achieve better cavity conformance. There are also five 6 French catheters that can house the radioactive source. One is located down the center of the device and the other 4 lumens are offset from the central catheter by 5 mm inside the balloon. These offset catheters allow dose modulation, and shaping of the irradiation dose to maximize target coverage while simultaneously minimizing unnecessary normal tissue irradiation. All the catheters are the same length and each have a radio-opaque plug at the distal end. Additionally, catheter 1 has a radio-opaque marker along the length of the catheter. Similar to the MammoSite the central channel houses a rigid insertion tool to allow for placement of the device that when removed permits the flexible stem comfortable approximation to the body.

Surgical insertion is performed in the same manner as the MammoSitedevice. Due to the multiple lumens in this device, the diameter of the shaft is slightly larger than the MammoSite,thus requiring a slightly larger incision.

Dosimetric constraints for the device mimic the MammoSite criteria with some additional recommendations and are shown in Table 2. SenoRx recommends a V95 of 95% with V150 < 50 cc and V200 < 10 cc, and a maximum skin dose of 125% of the prescribed dose.

Table 3. Contura size chart

Contura 4-5 balloon		Contura 4.5-6 balloon	
Volume (cc)	Diameter (mm)	Volume (cc)	Diameter (mm)
28	38	40	40
31	39	42	41
33	40	44	42
35	41	47	43
37	42	49	44
39	43	51	45
41.5	44	54	46
44	45	57	47
46.5	46	59	48
49.5	47	63	49
52	48	66	50
55	49	69	51
58	50	73	52
61.5	51	77	53
64.5	52	80	54
		84	55
		88	56
		93	57
		96	58
		102	59
		108	60

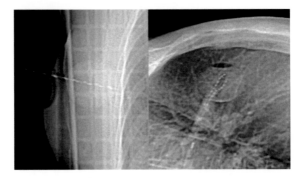

Figure 4.

When delivering an asymmetrical dose distribution, physicians and physicists must be vigilant to assure that treatment geometry exactly matches planned geometry. Therefore, daily quality assurance is very important and must not only verify the balloon integrity but also the position of the catheters.   White and black lines, offset by 180 degrees, are manufactured onto the Contura shaft. These are used, in conjunction with patient skin marks, to assure correct rotational orientation of catheter treatment position relative to planning position. Balloon integrity can be verified through orthogonal x-rays, CT scan, or ultrasound (Figure 4). Additionally, the shaft is marked along its length in order to quickly and easily check for any motion of the device in or out of the breast.

Eight month follow-up demonstrated similar toxicity and superior dose distribution to skin and ribs compared to the MammoSite®[33].Contura has been shown in increase the number of women eligible for APBI due to the ability of the vacuum port to remove fluid/air that would otherwise cause poor balloon/cavity conformance and require removal of the device [34].

1.2.5.3 SAVI

The Strut-Adjusted Volume Implant (SAVI) is also a multi-catheter breast brachytherapy applicator, but the catheters sit directly against the tissue, rather than housed within a balloon. SAVI received 510(k) approval for breast brachytherapy in the United States in 2006. The device consists of a central catheter surrounded by 6, 8, or 10 peripheral catheters that expand to fit the lumpectomy cavity (Figure 5). Thereare four sizes of the SAVI to fit a variety of lumpectomy cavity volumes. The different size devices have a varying number of peripheral catheters to ensure dosing flexibility and the naming convention indicates the number of peripheral catheters. The 6-1Mini and 6-1 applicator both have one central catheter and 6 peripheral catheters. The 8-1 applicator has one central catheter with 8 peripheral catheters and the 10-1 has one central catheter with 10 peripheral catheters. The size of the devices from smallest to largest is: 6-1Mini, 6-1, 8-1, and 10-1. The increase in size refers to an increase in both length and diameter of the expanded portion of the device at the distal tip and also volume irradiated. Table 4shows a reference sizing chart to assist in selecting the correct device for the lumpectomy cavity. Each of the applicators permits loading of the central and all of the peripheral catheters, with the central catheter's length extending slightly further than that of the peripheral catheters. The catheters are similar to the Contura's, being an open 6 French design that allows connection to the HDR afterloader. Since SAVI has multiple catheters adjacent to the target area, and each catheter can be loaded independently, this device is able to provide highly conformal dose delivery similar to that of interstitial breast brachytherapy. The tradeoff for this conformity is that the juxtaposition of the catheters to tissue increases the V150 and V200 compared to the balloon devices. The SAVI device also includes permanent radio-opaque markers that are built into three of the peripheral catheters for identification on CT or orthogonal films. The anterior-posterior (AP) and lateral film in Figure 6 shows the markers. These markers help for quick localization on orthogonal films and also for catheter identification during treatment planning. The markers are located on catheter numbers 2, 4, and 6, with the smallest marker located just short of the distal tip of catheter number 2.

Table 4. SAVI size chart

Diameter				
		2-3 cm	3-4 cm	4-5 cm
	2-3 cm	SAVI 6-1 Mini	NA	NA
	3-4 cm	SAVI 6-1 Mini	SAVI 6-1 Mini	NA
Long	4-5 cm	SAVI 6-1 Mini	SAVI 6-1 Mini	SAVI 6-1
Axis	5-6 cm	SAVI 6-1	SAVI 6-1	SAVI 8-1
	6-7 cm	SAVI 6-1	SAVI 8-1	SAVI 8-1
	7-8 cm	SAVI 8-1	SAVI 10-1	SAVI 10-1

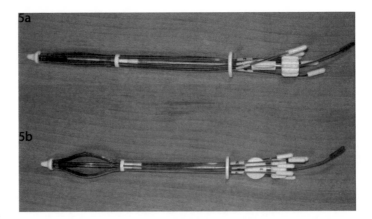

Figure 5.

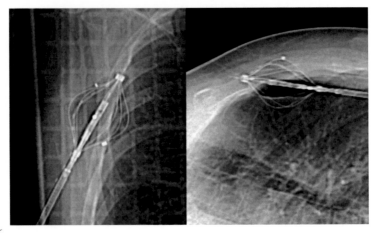

Figure 6.

Catheter number 4 has a medium sized marker located centrally and the largest marker is on catheter number 6, located proximally, just after the peripheral catheters start to separate from the central shaft.

The device comes with an expansion tool that slides down the central catheter and the device can be expanded or collapsed by holding the fixed hub at the base of the device and rotating the expansion tool. The device is introduced into the cavity in the collapsed form (Figure 5a) and then the expansion tool is turned clockwise to expand the device within the cavity (Figure 5b). The peripheral SAVI catheters createan outward pressure against the wall of the cavity and thus allow the appropriately sized SAVI to remain firmly in place. The expansion tool can be removed while not actively expanding or collapsing the device. Since the expansion tool is a rigid metal rod, removal gives greater flexibility to the device, and this flexibilityis similar to that of the MammoSite and Contura. However, it is recommended, that prior to each treatment, the expansion device is reinserted over the central catheter to allow for quick collapse and removal of the device in case of a radiation emergency.

Surgical insertion is similar to the other intracavitary devices, with the exception of instead of inflating the balloon, the device is opened with the use of the expansion tool. Additionally, due to the device's open cage-like configuration, seroma drainage can continue during the course of treatment and it is important to maintain clean wound dressings.

Dosimetric constraints for the device bridge those established by interstitial and MammoSite®brachytherapy[35] (Table 1). The guidelines suggest that 90% of the target volume (PTV_eval) should receive at least 90% of the dose (V90% > 90%) and that the volume of target tissue receiving 150% (V150) and 200% (V200) of the dose should remain less than 50 cc and 20 cc, respectively. These guidelines are usually easily achievable with a skin dose of ≤ 100% of the prescribed dose.

With extreme dose shaping, like interstitial brachytherapy, quality assurance is very important with the SAVI. Daily checks must be done to ensure that the planned treatment geometry is reproduced for the actual treatment delivery. Since this device is open in the center, it is not possible to visualize it well on ultrasound and therefore orthogonal x-rays or a CT scan must be used. The SAVI has marks along its length to check for in/out motion. The proximal hub is rigidly fixed and so it can also be used as a landmark, along with the skin, to check for in/out motion. Daily QA and device motion have been described by Scanderbeg et al [35].

The SAVI brachytherapy device has been shown to increase the patient population able to be treated by intracavitary APBI, and specifically in women with small breasts and/or tumorbeds close to the skin and/or chestwall. One study demonstrated an increase in patient eligibility by as much as 40%. This was accompanied by excellent dosimetry, cosmesis and outcome in these patients, although results are still preliminary [36]. Another published study compared SAVI to 3DCRT and MammoSite brachytherapy following NSABP B-39 guidelines and found lower doses to normal tissue (lung, skin and ribs) [37].

1.3. Summary

The three intracavitary devices have many similarities, such as their single-entry design, the surgical insertion, and dose and fractionation. However, there are small deviations with regards to dosimetric constraints and quality assurance practices. All the intracavitary devices require target coverage of at least 90% of the target covered by 90% of the dose. Several of the new APBI devices can now offer dosimetry that exceeds the traditional "acceptable" guidelines, originally established by MammoSite, and recommend V95 > 95%. Hotspot limitations are similar for the balloon devices with V150 < 50 cc for all devices and V200 < 10 cc for MammoSite and Contura and daily QA can be done with an ultrasound. Due to the strut/tissue approximation more closely resembling the interstitial implants the recommended V200 for SAVI is < 20 cc, with acceptable toxicity at 21 months follow-up. This difference is due to geometry of the devices. The balloon applicators displace the tissue away from the source and can have a lower overall V200 since the hotspot is kept within or at the surface of the balloon. However, this displacement of the struts from the tissue decreases somewhat the ability to modulate dose since by putting the catheters closer together and farther from the tissue being irradiated; it is more difficult to shape the dose. The SAVI device is similar to interstitial brachytherapy as it has struts that sit directly against the tissue. The proximity of the catheters to the target area means that the radiation dwell times in each location, to allow target dose at 1 cm, is relatively lower than in the balloon devices. Being close to the treated target area allows maximal dosing flexibility, second only to interstitial, with the tradeoff that tissue lying directly against the catheter is subject to higher local doses with typically higher V150 and V200. However, this juxtaposition mirrors interstitial brachytherapy and thus the V200 allowable is higher. As mentioned previously, it was demonstrated in two studies that tissue stretching caused by the expansion of the balloon effectively treated a larger margin. However, the variability between these two studies seems to indicate that the effect of tissue stretching on treatment volume may not be fixed. It may be a patient variable depending on breast tissue type, cavity volume, and balloon size. Tissue stretching has not been studied in either the Contura or the SAVI; although results from the Contura would be expected to behave similarly to the MammoSite®since they both have balloon applicators. Results from the SAVI remain to be seen, but if it does not stretch the tissue to the same extent as a balloon device then the clinician could possibly treat to a larger margin (within dosimetric constraints) or specifically choose a balloon device for higher risk patients, if these needs outweigh the needs to conform the dose to anatomical constraints.

1.4. Conclusions

The popularity of APBI is increasing, especially since the introduction of single-entry devices, even with the lack of published prospective data. Unless prospective randomized data demonstrate a much decreased local control or increased toxicity, it is likely that this trend will continue with more women choosing an accelerated course of treatment that spares more normal tissue.

Any method of breast cancer irradiation has its pros and cons, including each of the methods described in this chapter. The intracavitary devices each have their own advantages and disadvantages, and since most of the data coming on these devices is still immature, it may still be several years before clinicians have a clear answer as to what is best for a particular patient. However, most likely, a clinician will have to be stocked with a full arsenal of devices to best treat the unique specifications of a particular patient as every individual is different and calls for a unique, personal treatment. An oncoplastic procedure contraindicates an intracavitary device and so interstitial or external therapy must be used if a patient desires APBI. If a patient has a very small skin bridge or close approximation to rib, heart and lung (even simultaneously), then the SAVI device provides the greater dosing flexibility; and if a patient has a non-irregular shaped cavity in the center of the breast, a single-source MammoSite is the easiest and fastest method of treatment, with the greatest body of mature literature. If the balloon devices do compress tissue more than the strut devices, and the strut cannot be safely used to treat an equivalent amount of tissue, the risk of the patient may guide the device selection. In addition the ability of the ultrasound for use as QA, rather than time in the simulator for orthogonal X-rays or a CT scan may be important in some clinics. In any case, it behooves the clinician and physicist to be familiar and comfortable with all the tools at their disposal in order to properly provide the best breast cancer care for a patient.

Abbreviations

WBI	whole breast irradiation
ABPI	accelerated partial breast irradiation
SAVI	*Strut Adjusted Volume Implant*
3DCRT	3 dimensional conformal radiotherapy
IORT	intraoperative radiation therapy
HDR	high-dose-rate
LDR	low-dose-rate
NCI	National Cancer Institute
NSABP	National Surgical Adjuvant Breast and Bowel Project
ABS	American Brachytherapy Society
ASBS	American Society of Breast Surgeons
ASTRO	American Society for Therapeutic Radiology and Oncology
Vxx	Volume of tissue receiving xx% of the prescribed dose

References

[1] Veronesi, U; Cascinelli, N; Mariani, L; *et al.*Twenty-year follow-up of a randomized study comparing breast-conserving surgery with radical mastectomy for early breast cancer. *N Engl J Med*, 2002, 347(16), 1227-1232.

[2] Fisher, B; Anderson, S; Bryant, J; *et al.* Twenty-year follow-up of a randomized trial comparing total mastectomy, lumpectomy, and lumpectomy plus irradiation for the treatment of invasive breast cancer. *N Engl J Med*, 2002, 347(16), 1233-1241.

[3] Clarke, M; Collins, R; Darby, S;*et al.* Effects of radiotherapy and of differences in the extent of surgery for early breast cancer on local recurrence and15-year survival: an overview of the randomised trials. *Lancet*, 2005, 366(9503), 2087-2106.

[4] Fowble, B. Ipsilateral breast tumor recurrence following breast-conserving surgery for early-stage invasive cancer. *Acta Oncol*, 1999, 38 Suppl 13, 9-17.

[5] Fowble, B; Solin, LJ; Schultz, DJ;*et al.*Breast recurrence following conservative surgery and radiation: patterns of failure, prognosis, and pathologic findings from mastectomy specimens with implications for treatment. *Int J Radiat Oncol Biol Phys.*, 1990, 19(4), 833-842.

[6] Ott, OJ; Hildebrandt, G; Potter, R; *et al.*Accelerated partial breast irradiation with multi-catheterbrachytherapy: Local control, side effects and cosmetic outcome for 274 patients. Results of the German-Austrian multi-centre trial. *Radiother Oncol*, 2007, 82(3), 281-286.

[7] Vicini, FA; Arthur, DW. Breast brachytherapy: North American experience. *Semin Radiat Oncol*, 2005, 15(2), 108-115.

[8] Arthur, DW; Winter, K; Kuske, RR; *et al.* A Phase II trial of brachytherapy alone after lumpectomy for select breast cancer: tumor control and survival outcomes of RTOG 95-17. *Int J Radiat Oncol Biol Phys.*, 2008, 72(2), 467-473.

[9]   King, TA; Bolton, JS; Kuske, RR;*et al.* Long-term results of wide-field brachytherapy as the sole method of radiation therapy after segmental mastectomy for T(is,1,2) breast cancer. *Am J Surg.*, 2000, 180(4), 299-304.

[10] Polgar, C; Sulyok, Z; Fodor, J; *et al.*Sole brachytherapy of the tumor bed after conservative surgery for T1 breast cancer: five-year results of a phase I-II study and initial findings of a randomized phase III trial. *J Surg Oncol*, 2002, 80(3), 121-128, discussion 129.

[11] Polgar, C; Fodor, J; Major, T; *et al.*Breast-conserving treatment with partial or whole breast irradiation for low-risk invasive breast carcinoma--5-year results of a randomized trial. *Int J Radiat Oncol Biol Phys.*, 2007, 69(3), 694-702.

[12] Arthur, DW; Vicini, FA; Kuske, RR;*et al.* Accelerated partial breast irradiation: an updated report from the American Brachytherapy Society. *Brachytherapy*, 2003, 2(2), 124-130.

[13] Smith, BD; Arthur, DW; Buchholz, TA; *et al.* Accelerated partial breast irradiation consensus statement from the American Society for Radiation Oncology (ASTRO). *Int J Radiat Oncol Biol Phys.*, 2009, 74(4), 987-1001.

[14] Baglan, KL; Sharpe, MB; Jaffray, D; *et al.*Accelerated partial breast irradiation using 3D conformal radiation therapy (3D-CRT).*Int J Radiat Oncol Biol Phys.*, 2003, 55(2), 302-11.

[15] Vicini, FA; Chen, P; Wallace, M; *et al.* Interim cosmetic results and toxicity using 3D conformal external beam radiotherapy to deliver accelerated partial breast irradiation in patients with early-stage breast cancer treated with breast-conserving therapy. *Int J Radiat Oncol Biol Phys.*, 2007, 69(4), 1124-1130.

[16] Recht, A; Ancukiewicz, M; Alm El-Din, MA; *et al.* Lung Dose-Volume Parameters and the Risk of Pneumonitis for Patients Treated With Accelerated Partial-Breast Irradiation Using Three-Dimensional Conformal Radiotherapy. *J Clin Oncol*, 2009, 27(24), 3887-3893.

[17] Hepel, JT; Tokita, M; Macausland, SG; *et al.*Toxicity of Three-Dimensional Conformal Radiotherapy for Accelerated Partial Breast Irradiation. *Int J Radiat Oncol Biol Phys.*, 2009, 75(5), 1290-1296.

[18] Livi, L; Buonamici, FB; Simontacchi, G;*et al.*Accelerated partial breast irradiation with IMRT: new technical approach and interim analysis of acute toxicity in a phase III randomized clinical trial. *Int J Radiat Oncol Biol Phys*, article in press, 2009.

[19] Intra, M; Leonardi, C; Luini, A; *et al.*Full-dose intraoperative radiotherapy with electrons in breast surgery: broadening the indications. *Arch Surg.*, 2005, 140(10), 936-939.

[20] Mussari, S; Sabino Della Sala, W; Busana, L; *et al.*Full-dose intraoperative radiotherapy with electrons in breast cancer. First report on late toxicity and cosmetic results from a single-institution experience. *Strahlenther Onkol*, 2006, 182(10), 589-595.

[21] Pignol, JP; Rakovitch, E; Keller, BM;*et al.* Tolerance and acceptance results of a palladium-103 permanent breast seed implant Phase I/II study. *Int J Radiat Oncol Biol Phys.*, 2009, 73(5), 1482-1488.

[22] Keller, BM; Pignol, JP; Rakovitch, E; *et al.* A radiation badge survey for family members living with patients treated with a (103)Pd permanent breast seed implant. *Int J Radiat Oncol Biol Phys.*, 2008, 70(1), 267-271.

[23] Benitez, PR; Keisch, ME; Vicini, F; *et al.* Five-year results: the initial clinical trial of MammoSite balloon brachytherapy for partial breast irradiation in early-stage breast cancer. *Am J Surg.*, 2007, 194(4), 456-462.

[24] Vicini, F; Beitsch, P; Quiet, C; *et al.* Two year analysis of treatment efficacy and cosmesis by the American Society of Breast Surgeons (ASBS) MammoSite Breast Brachytherapy Registry Trial in patients treated with accelerated partial breast irradiation (APBI). *J Clin Oncol*, 2006, 18, S529.

[25] Cuttino, LW; Keisch, M; Jenrette, JM; *et al.* Multi-institutional experience using the MammoSite radiation therapy system in the treatment of early-stage breast cancer: 2-year results. *Int J Radiat Oncol Biol Phys.*, 2008, *71(1)*, 107-114.

[26] Prestidge, B; Sadeghi, A; Rosenthal, A; al. e. Local control of early stage breast cancer using MammoSite HDR brachytherapy. *Int J Radiat Oncol Biol Phys.*, 2006, 66, S215.

[27] Chao, KK; Vicini, FA; Wallace, M; *et al.*Analysis of treatment efficacy, cosmesis, and toxicity using the MammoSite breast brachytherapy catheter to deliver accelerated partial-breast irradiation: the William Beaumont hospital experience. *Int J Radiat Oncol Biol Phys.*, 2007, 69(1), 32-40.

[28] Keisch, M; Vicini, F; Kuske, RR; *et al.*Initial clinical experience with the MammoSite breast brachytherapy applicator in women with early-stage breast cancer treated with breast-conserving therapy. *Int J Radiat Oncol Biol Phys.*, 2003, 55(2), 289-293.

[29] Nelson, JC; Beitsch, PD; Vicini, FA; *et al.* Four-year clinical update from the American Society of Breast Surgeons MammoSite brachytherapy trial. *Am J Surg.*, 2009, 198(1), 83-91.

[30] Dickler, A; Kirk, M; Choo, J; *et al.* Treatment volume and dose optimization of the MammoSite breast brachytherapy applicator. *Int J Radiat Oncol Biol Phys.*, 2004, 59, 469-474.

[31] Edmondson, G; Vicini, F; Chen, P; *et al.* Dosimetric characteristics of the MammoSite RTS, a new breast applicator. *Int J Radiat Oncol Biol Phys.*, 2002, 52, 1132-1139.

[32] Cuttino, LW; Todor, D; Rosu, M; Arthur, DW. Skin and chest wall dose with multi-catheter and MammoSite breast brachytherapy: Implications for late toxicity. *Brachytherapy*, 2009, 8(2), 223-226.

[33] Brown, S; McLaughlin, M; Pope, K; Haile, K; Hughes, L; Israel, PZ. Initial radiation experience evaluating early tolerance and toxicities in patients undergoing accelerated partial breast irradiation using the Contura Multi-Lumen Balloon breast brachytherapy catheter. *Brachytherapy*, 2009, 8(2), 227-233.

[34] Wilder, RB; Curcio, LD; Khanijou, RK; *et al.* A Contura catheter offers dosimetric advantages over a MammoSite catheter that increase the applicability of accelerated partial breast irradiation. *Brachytherapy*, 2009, 8(4), 373-378.

[35] Scanderbeg, DJ; Yashar, C; Rice, R;*et al.* Clinical implementation of a new HDR brachytherapy device for partial breast irradiation. *Radiother Oncol*, 2009, 90(1), 36-42.

[36] Yashar, C; Blair, S; Wallace, A; *et al.* Initial Clinical Experience with the strut assisted volume implant brachytherapy applicator for accelerated partial breast irradiation. *Brachytherapy*, 2009, *8(4)*, 367-372.

[37] Scanderbeg, D; Yashar, C; White, G; *et al.* Evaluation of three APBI techniques under NSABP B-39 guidelines. *J Appl Clin Med Phys.*, 2010, 11(1), 274-280.

In: Brachytherapy
Editor: Leoni M. Fische

Chapter 6

Innovative Use of Balloon Applicators for Gynecological High Dose Rate Brachytherapy

Susan Richardson and W. Perry Grigsby
Washington University School of Medicine &
the Mallinckrodt Institute of Radiology, Saint Louis, Missouri, USA

Abstract

Introduction

The use of balloon brachytherapy devices for High Dose Rate (HDR) partial breast irradiation is well established. Alternatively, balloon applicators can be used for HDR brachytherapy treatment of gynecological malignancies. This includes treatment for (1) post operative endometrial cancer and (2) inoperable endometrial cancer.Here, we describe the clinical and dosimetric methodology for these two treatment sites.

Materials and Methods

Balloon devices were used as applicators for vaginal vault irradiation for patients treated post-operatively and for treatment of the uterusfor those with inoperable endometrial cancer. Patients were treated with a Varian iX Ir-192 high dose rate brachytherapy source.Three dimensional treatment planning was done with BrachyVision 8.2 and was based on CT scans acquired for each treatment fraction.

Results

For irradiation of the vaginal vault, the use of a balloon applicator reduces the frequency of air gaps between the vaginal mucosa and the applicator as compared to a standard segmented cylinder applicator.It provides excellent radiation dose coverage of the target area with acceptable doses to the bladder and the rectum.For treatment of the uterine serosa, the dose distribution is similar to that obtained through the use of Simon-Heyman capsules while maintaining the ease of a single-entry applicator. It also provides a more reproducible treatment because the volume of the balloon is easily duplicated from fraction to fraction.The insertion and removal of the applicator in both treatment sites is well tolerated.

Conclusion

The use of balloon applicators in gynecological sites is a clinically feasible and safe method of patient treatment.Balloon applicators offer the simplicity of a single-entry, single channel tool. The applicator itself is patient specific based on the fill volume of the balloon and can be the same from fraction to fraction, or can adapt if the patient anatomy changes.The dose distributions obtained are similar to conventional treatment devices.Other treatment sites may also benefit from the use of a balloon applicator.

Introduction

A wide variety of applicators exist for the High Dose Rate (HDR) brachytherapy treatment of gynecological malignancies.For post-operative endometrial cancer, the most commonly used device, according to a survey done by the American Brachytherapy Society, is a standard segmented cylinder. [1] For inoperable endometrial cancer, a wide variety of devices are used including a single channel intrauterine tandem, Heyman capsules [2, 3], Bauer applicators, and the Rotte Y applicator [4-7]. All of these devices are acceptable for the treatment of gynecological malignancies; however, alternative devices such as a balloon applicator may offer distinct advantages.The clinical and dosimetric methodology of using a balloon applicator for treatment of both post-operative and inoperable endometrial cancer will be discussed.

Materials and Methods

Applicator Insertion

At our institution, gynecologic brachytherapy is administered in 6 weekly fractions. A Mammosite® (Cytyc Corp., Marlborough, MA) breast brachytherapy balloon catheter is used as the applicator.The Mammosite® balloon is well described in the literature for delivery of partial breast brachytherapy and will not be discussed here. [8-10]The procedure for use of this balloon technique for gynecologic patients has been termed GynSite®. Patients are brought to our brachytherapy suite and placed in the dorsal lithotomy position.Gold markers are placed at the cervical os or vaginal apex. The deflated applicator in inserted into either the vagina for vaginal cuff brachytherapy, or into the cervical os for treatment of the uterine serosa. The insertion of the balloon in this manner is an off-label use of the device. The balloon is inflated until resistance is felt with a 5% Conray and normal saline solution.The balloon fill volume is then documented. Patients have a Foley catheter placed in the bladder.

CT simulation is done on a Philips Brilliance scanner with 3 mm slice resolution (Philips Medical, Chesterfield, MO).

Treatment Planning and Treatment

Three dimensional treatment planning is performed with Varian BrachyVision 8.2 (Varian Medical Systems, Palo Alto, CA).Organs at risk including the bladder and rectum are contoured.The balloon catheter is digitized and potential dwell positions are marked every 0.5 cm.The treatment plans are optimized to deliver the prescribed dose to the surface of the balloon.For treatment of the vaginal apex, we deliver 400 to 700 cGy per fraction for 6 fractions depending on stage and whether or not the patient is receiving external beam radiotherapy.For treatment of the uterine serosa, prescriptions are 600 to 800 cGy per fraction for 6 fractions, again depending on clinical factors.Patients are treated with a Varian iX afterloaded Ir-192 source. After completion of each treatment, the balloon is deflated and removed. The balloon is sterilized and reused for the patient's remaining fractions.

Most patients received concurrent intensity modulated external beam radiotherapy(IMRT) to treat both the target and lymph nodes.Brachytherapy typically takes place one day a week while external beam radiotherapy is administered 4 days a week.

Discussion

Post Operative Endometrial Brachytherapy

Several studies have shown that although most institutions use a single channel vaginal cylinder for post operative endometrial brachytherapy, there are problems with the conformance of vaginal surface to the applicator.Each patient has unique anatomy that depends on the patient's age, parity, hormonal status, and post-hysterectomy surgical technique.It has been determined that in many patients air gaps exist around the cylinder, resulting in reduced dose to the vaginal mucosa. Cameron, et al. found that in a study of 25 patients, there were a total of 37 air gaps found on the patient's first fraction CT scan. [11] A subsequent study by our group investigated the rate of air gap occurrence on multiple fraction CT scans. [12]In summary, we found that in 25 patients, a total of 90 air gaps were identified in 150 procedures (60%).Some patients had an air gap in the same physical region of their vagina over all fractions of their treatment and some had sporadic air gaps.The average dose reduction to the vaginal mucosa surface in the region of the air gap was 27%. An example of one patient's very large air gap is shown in Figure 1.

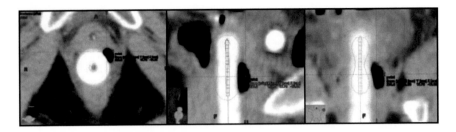

Figure 1. Axial, coronal, and sagittal views of a patient with a large air gap occurring with treatment with a standard vaginal cylinder for vaginal apex brachytherapy.

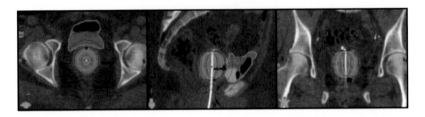

Figure 2. Use of a balloon applicator for high dose rate irradiation of the vaginal apex.

Vaginal apex brachytherapy is sometimes the only radiation therapy an endometrial cancer patient receives. Air gaps can cause an under-dose of the target which could potentially lead to relapse. Additionally, a lack of conformance could allow the applicator to move inside the vagina. A more patient specific applicator could help eliminate air gaps, thereby improving the dosimetry, reducing applicator motion, and being more comfortable and tolerable to patient. Because of these findings, alternative applicators, such as a balloon, that has the potential to be more conformal to the patient's anatomy, were investigated. Cylinders are available only in discrete sizes (2, 2.5 cm diameter, etc.) whereas a balloon has different shapes (spherical or elliptical) and continuously variable fill volumes (35cc – 125cc).Therefore, a balloon could allow a more patient-specific delivery of the radiation to thevaginal apex. An example of a patient treatment with the use of a balloon applicator for high dose rate irradiation of the vaginal apex is shown in Figure 2.

Thirty consecutive patients were treated with an intra-vaginal balloon in our department. A summary of all patient specific parameters can be found in Miller,*et al*. [13]. The mean fill volume of the balloon was 47.3 cc. The mean 2cc bladder dose was 48.6% of the prescribed dose and the average 2cc rectal dose was 71.1% of the prescribed dose. There were no acute grade 3 or 4 complications and all insertions were tolerated well with minimal medication. All patients completed treatment. We concluded that the intra-vaginal balloon technique provided a safe method for anatomically conformal brachytherapy vaginal cuff irradiation.

A direct dosimetric comparison was also done in 20 patients treated with either an intra-vaginal balloon or a vaginal cylinder. Ten consecutive patients treated with each device were retrospectively analyzed for air gap formation and for doses to the organs at risk. Out of the ten patients (6 fractions each) treated with a vaginal cylinder, 19 air gaps were found.For the ten patients treated with an intra-vaginal balloon (6 fractions each), only 2 air gaps were found. [14] The target dose in the regions of the air gap averaged 70% and 82% of the prescribed dose for the cylinder and balloon, respectively. This indicates that the air gaps are smaller in size have smaller dosimetric impact when using the balloon applicator. The doses to the bladder and rectum for the two applicators in this study are summarized below in Table 1.

In general, the use of a balloon applicator increased the delivered dose to the 2cc of bladder and 2cc of rectum. This is understandable because the diameter of an inserted balloon is greater than a typical cylinder diameter (4 cm vs. 2.5 cm) and pushes more on the internal organs with inflation. However, the work of Miller, *et al.* indicates that these doses are clinically acceptable with no acute Grade 3 or 4 side effects in our patient population.

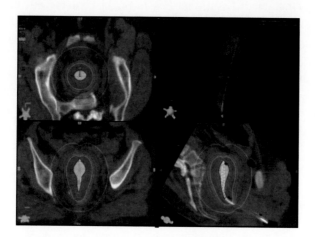

Figure 3. Upper left and lower panels show the 2D projections of the balloon in the uterus and the dose distribution. The upper right panel shows the prescription isodose cloud as a red color wash.

**Table 1. Doses and standard deviations for bladder and rectum
treated with balloon and cylinder applicators.
Numbersare given as a percentage of the prescribed dose**

Dose to OAR as a % of Prescribed Dose	Rectum		Bladder	
	Balloon	Cylinder	Balloon	Cylinder
2cc	70.1 +/- 5	57.9 +/- 5	45.1 +/- 5	34.7 +/- 10
Mean Dose	27.7 +/- 4	23.4 +/- 3	36.9 +/- 5	18.0 +/- 5
Max Dose	102.5 +/- 19	90.8 +/- 9	79.6 +/- 9	57.8 +/- 16

Inoperable Endometrial Cancer

A small percentage of endometrial cancer patients (3-9%) are not surgical candidates due to obesity or other medical conditions and depend on radiotherapy treatment alone. [15-17] Excellent local control has been reported for inoperable patients in several studies. [18, 19] Though a wide variety of applicators have been used for the treatment of this disease, manufacturer and training support for some (such as Heyman capsules) is diminishing.While using a single channel tandem is thought to be the most convenient and easiest mechanism for treatment, it does not produce an ideal dose distribution. Mock, *et al.*reported that on average, single channel applicators only covered 47% of the uterus while multi-channel Heyman applications covered 70%. [20] The use of a balloon applicator may be able to produce a better dose distribution while maintaining the insertion and planning ease of a single channel device. Figure 3 shows the use of a balloon applicator in the uterus for treatment of inoperable endometrial cancer.

When compared with other treatment devices, the use of an intra-uterine balloon produces a distribution that is more similar to that of Heyman capsules rather than tandem alone. The use of a tandem alone limits the amount of dose that can be safely delivered because of the large amount of tissue that lies in direct contact with the applicator. When using Heyman capsules, usually multiple capsules (3+) are inserted for treatment. Each capsule and source channel can share in the contribution of the prescribed dose. Subsequently, the uterus can be covered by a higher isodose line. [20] Similarly, the use of a balloon applicator allows the tissue to be pushed away from the source and source channel and increases the depth dose across the uterus as shown in Figure 3. Therefore, the dose distribution can be tailored to push dose laterally and with increased dose at the fundus compared to a tandem.

Though Heyman capsules allow flexibility in dose tailoring, the insertion of 5-7 capsules throughout the course of the patient's treatment may prove to be difficult with changing anatomy. Since we deliver brachytherapy concurrently with external beam radiotherapy, anatomical changes are common and usually involve the uterus decreasing in size. A balloon device is easy to insert and remove without requiring heavy sedation, even after many treatment fractions. Treatment planning is also simplified compared to multi-channel insertions of Heyman capsules since a balloon applicator has only a single channel. Additionally, the fraction-to-fraction reproducibility of a Heyman capsule implant is difficult. With a balloon applicator, the fill volume is documented and easy to duplicate with each subsequent fraction.

To date, we have treated 4 patients with an intra-uterine balloon applicator for treatment of inoperable endometrial cancer. None of the patients treated with an intra-uterine balloon experienced any thrombo-embolic events within the first 30 days after treatment. None of the patients experienced any acute toxicity from device insertion, removal, or administration of the treatment.

Conclusions

For post operative endometrial cancer, the use of an intra-vaginal balloon delivers a dose distribution similar to that of the standard segmented cylinder with moderate dose increases to the organs at risk. This flexibility allows the device to better conform to the patient's anatomy thus reducing air gaps between the applicator and the vaginal mucosa. The use of a balloon applicator reduced the air gap formation from 1 in 3 with a cylinder to 1 in 30 with a balloon. [14] This can increase the dose to the target lymphatic channels and potentially improve survival.

Inoperable endometrial cancer is difficult to treat due to patient morbidity (and usually) obesity. The use of a multiple channel applicator produces a more desirable dose distribution than a single channel applicator. However, they are more complicated to insert and require more labor intensive treatment planning. Additionally, due to changes in the patient's anatomy over the course of treatment, the insertion of multiple channel devices may not be possible after a few fractions. The use of a balloon applicator retains the ease of use of a single channel device, but produces dose distributions that are more similar to that of a multiple channel applicator.

References

[1]   Nag, S; Erickson, B; Parikh, S; et al. The American Brachytherapy Society recommendations for high-dose-rate brachytherapy for carcinoma of the endometrium. *IntJRadiatOncolBiolPhys.*, 2000, 48, 779-790.

[2]   Andersen, WA; Peters, WA; Fechner, RE; et al. Radiotherapeutic alternatives to standard management of adenocarcinoma of the endometrium. *GynecolOncol*, 1983,16, 383-92.

[3]   Landgren, RC; Fletcher, GH; Delclos, L; et al. Irradiation of endometrial cancer in patients with medical contraindications to surgery or unresectable lesions. *AmJRadio*, 11976, 126, 148- 54.

[4]   Gerszten, K; Faul, C; Kelley, J; et al. Twice-daily high-dose-rate brachytherapy for medically inoperable uterine cancer, *Brachytherapy*, 2006, 5, 118-121.

[5]   Bauer, M; Schulz-Wendtland, R. A new afterloading applicator for primary brachytherapy of endometrial cancer, *SELECTRON Brachyther J (Suppl*,1991, 2, 56- 58.

[6]   Nori, D; Hilaris, B; Anderson, L; et al. A new endometrial applicator, *Int J Radiat Oncol Biol Phys.*,1982, 8, 941-945.

[7]   Rotte, K; Schneider, J. Technique and results of HDR afterloading in cancer of the endometrium. In: A. Martinez, C. Orton and R. Mould, Editors, Brachytherapy HDR and LDR, *Nucletron Corp.*, Columbia, MD,1990, 68-79.

[8]   Keisch, M; Vicini, F; Kuske, RR; et al. Initial clinical experience with the MammoSite breast brachytherapy applicator in women with early-stage breast cancer treated with breastconserving therapy. *Int J Radiat Oncol Biol Phys.*, 2003, 55, 289-293.

[9]   Edmundson, G; Vicini, FA; Chen, PY; et al. Dosimetric characteristics of the MammoSite RTS, a new breast brachytherapy applicator. *Int J Radiat Oncol Biol Phys.*, 2002, 52, 1132-1139.

[10] Streeter, O; Vicini, F; Keisch, M; et al.MammoSite® radiation therapy system. *The Breast*, 2003, 12, 491-496.

[11] Cameron, AL; Cornes, P; Al-Booz, H. Brachytherapy in endometrial cancer: Quantification of air pockets around a vaginal cylinder. *Brachytherapy*, 2008, 7, 355- 358.

[12] Richardson, S; Palaniswaamy, G; Grigsby, PW. Dosimetric effects of air pockets around high-dose rate brachytherapy vaginal cylinders.*Int J Radiat Oncol Biol Phys.*, 2010, (in press).

[13] Miller, DA; Richardson, S; Grigsby, PW. A new method of anatomicallyconformal vaginal cuff HDR brachytherapy. *Gynecol Oncol*, 2010, 116(3), 413-418.

[14] Richardson, S; Grigsby, PW. Dosimetric evaluation of the gynsite device for vaginal apex irradiation. *Med Phys.*, 2009, 36(6), 2773-2774.

[15] Patanaphan, V; Salazer, OM; Chougule, P. What can be expected when radiation therapy becomes the only curative alternative for endometrial cancer? *Cancer*, 1985, 55, 1462-1467.

[16] Taghian, A; Pernot, M; Hoffstetter, S; et al. Radiation therapy alone for medically inoperable patients with adenocarcinoma of the endometrium. *Int J Radiat Oncol Biol Phys.*, 1988, 15, 1135-1140.

[17] Rouanet, P; Dubois, JB; Gely, S; Pourquier, H. Exclusive radiation therapy in endometrial carcinoma. *Int J Radiat Oncol Biol Phys.*, 1993, 26, 223-228.

[18] Rose,PG; Baker,S; Kern,M; et al., Primary radiation therapy for endometrial carcinoma: A case controlled study,*Int J Radiat Oncol Biol Phys.*, 1993, 27, 585-590.

[19] Coon, D; Beriwal, S; Heron, DE; et al.High-Dose-Rate Rotte 'Y' Applicator Brachytherapy for Definitive Treatment of Medically Inoperable Endometrial Cancer: 10-Year Results, *Int J Radiat Oncol Biol Phys.*, 2008, 71, 779-783.

[20] Mock, M; Knocke, T; Fellner, C; Pötter, R. Analysis of different application systems and CT-controlled planning variant in the treatment of primary endometrial carcinomas. Is brachytherapy treatment of the entire uterus technically possible? *Strahlenther Onkol*, 1998, Jun, 174(6), 320-8.

In: Brachytherapy
Editor: Leoni M. Fische

Chapter 7

Brachytherapy in Thailand: Summary of Reports

Viroj Wiwanitkit
Wiwanikit House, Bangkhae, Bangkok, Thailand

Abstract

Brachytherapy is an important cancer therapy modality. The common cancers for which this kind of therapy is useful include skin cancer, prostate cancer, cervical cancer,etc. This kind of treatment has been used in Thailand for a long time, and many reports on this cancer treatment have been done there. In this specific article, the author summarizes the important reports on brachytherapy in Thailand. Special focus is placed on types, dosing and side effects.

Introduction to Brachytherapy

Brachytherapy, by term, means the therapy at near distance. Normally, this term is used in oncology for describing a method of cancer treatment that is based on near distance destruction of a tumor cell. At present, brachytherapy is an important cancer therapy modality. The common cancers for which this kind of therapy is useful include skin cancer, prostate cancer, cervical cancer,etc. This kind of treatment has been used for a long time. At first, the use of a radioactive substance was the main theme for brachytherapy. However, at present, new approaches such as using electricity and nanomaterialshas become the new challenge for brachytherapy.

In general, brachytherapy is an activity in the radiotherapy section of a hospital. This is usually done at a large hospital with available facilities. At least, the setting must have the ability to keep control of usage of a radioactive substance. The setting must also havea specific ward and apparatus for applying brachytherapy to the patients.

Brachytherapy in Thailand

Brachytherapy has been usedin Thailand for a long time, and many reports on this cancer treatment have been done there. Historically, brachytherapy was first used in Thailand in the largest hospital, Siriraj Hospital. This was a long time ago. After that, brachytherapy came into general use in many tertiary hospitals of Thailand. However, presently there are only a few brachytherapy centers in Thailand and very few practitioners who are experts in this area. In this specific article, the author hereby summarizes the important reports on brachytherapy in Thailand. Special focus is placed on types, dosing and side effects.

**Table 1. Interesting reports on brachytherapy
for cervical cancer in Thailand**

Authors	Details
Wangwiwat [1]	This is the early paper describing the brachytherapy in Thailand in its first phase in the past half century [1].
Tungsubutra [2]	This is another early paper describing brachytherapy in Thailand [2]. The review is by a famous Thai radiologist at that time [2].
Tungsubutra [3]	Tungsubutra assessed on the role of a PC. in treatment planning and dosimetry in teletherapy, brachytherapy and combined teletherapy and brachytherapy in the management of carcinoma of the cervix in Thailand [3].
Kongthanarat [4]	Kongthanarat reported on a five-year result and complications with high-dose rate after loading brachytherapy in cervix cancer using a straight tandem in a Thai tertiary hospital [4]. Kongthanarat showed that a simple linear source arrangement for high-dose rate brachytherapy could be safely and effectively used in the supplementary treatment of carcinoma of the uterine cervix [4].
Raruen [5]	Raruen performed an analysis of point a dose in patients with cervical cancer treated with high dose rate brachytherapy [5]. Raruen concluded that "For roughly planning, with dose rate of 5 Gy per fraction at point A, TRAK exponent 2 about 0.37 cGy at 1 meter can be used with satisfactory [5]."
Pairatchvet et al. [6]	Pairatchvet et al. studied the high-dose-rate interstitial brachytherapy in the management of carcinoma of the uterine cervix and other gynecologic malignancies and reported that "This technique is feasible, providing good local control without serious complications. However, long term follow-up is needed [6]."
Seenukhroah [7]	Seenukhroah reported on a verification of absorbed dose in muscle values calculated by the brachyvision software for the treatment planning of carcinoma of cervix using iridium-192 intracavitary insertion technique in a tertiary hospital in Thailand [7].
Peesee et al. [8]	Raemsiri et al. reported on low dose rate brachytherapy caesium-137 afterloading in the treatment of carcinoma of uterine cervix focusing on resulted acturial survival rate [8].
Lorvidhaya et al. [9]	Lorvidhaya et al. reported on high-dose-rate afterloading brachytherapy in carcinoma of the cervix [9]. A favorable experience of 1992 patients was presented in this specific report [9].

**Table 2. Interesting reports on brachytherapy for
prostate cancer in Thailand**

Authors	Details
Pattaranutaporn [10]	Pattaranutaporn reported on Iridium-192 wax mould therapy for the treatment of superfical tumor of the floor of the mouth [10].
Patjanasoontorn et al. [11]	Patjanasoontorn et al. reported on the high-dose-rate endobronchial brachytherapy for the local control of intraluminal bronchogenic carcinoma [11]. Patjanasoontorn et al. reached the conclusion that "The procedures are well tolerated and are relatively less expensive than other endobronchial palliative treatments [11]."
Panichevaluket al. [12]	Panichevaluket al. studied on theintracavitary HDR 60 Brachytherapy in the nasopharyngeal cancer and reported that this approach can be a good alternative for treatment of nasopharyngeal cancer [12].

1. Reports on Brachytherapy for Cervical Cancer in Thailand

Of several cancers in females, the most common cancer is cervical cancer. Cervical cancer'scorrelation to the human papilloma virus (HPV) infection has already been proven. This infection is still highly prevalent among Thai women and can be the cause of the high prevalence of cervical cancer in Thailand. The practice of brachytherapy in Thailand was first introduced for treatment of cervical cancer. Hence, the reports on brachytherapy for cervical cancer can be more available than those on other cancers (Table 1).

2. Reports on Brachytherapy for Skin Cancer in Thailand

Skin cancer can be seen in Thailand but it is not common. The main therapeutic option for treatment of skin cancer is the surgical approach. The use of brachytherapy is limited. However, there is no officical publication on brachytherapy for skin cancer in Thailand.

3. Reports on Bachytherapy for Prostate Cancer in Thailand

Prostate cancer is a common cancer of the male genital tract. This cancer can be seen in Thailand, similar to other countries. The main treatment option for this cancer is the surgical approach. However, there are also other additional alternatives including hormonal therapy and brachytherapy. However, there is no officical publication on brachytherapy for skin cancer in Thailand.

4. Reports on Bachytherapy for Other Cancers in Thailand

The usage of brachytherapy for other cancers is limited. However, there are some official reports on this topic as quoted in Table 2.

References

[1]   Wangwiwat, D. Treatment of cervical cancer with Fletcher's applicator and deep irradiation. *J Int Coll Surg Thai.*, 1961, 4(1), 48-56.

[2]   Tungsubutra, K. Recent advances in radiation therapy of uterine cervical cancer. *ThaiJRadiol*, 1984, 30(1), 61-67.

[3]   Tungsubutra, K. Assessment of the role of a PC in treatment planning and dosimetry in teletherapy, brachytherapy and combined teletherapy and brachytherapy in the management of carcinoma of the cervix in Thailand, *Thai J Radiol*, 1984, 30(1), 45-50.

[4]   Kongthanarat, Y. Five-year result and complications with high-dose rate after loading brachytherapy in cervix cancer using a straight tandem. *J Rajvithi Hosp*, 1997, 7(3), 39-46.

[5]   Raruen, S. Analysis of point a dose in patients with cervical cancer treated with high dose rate brachytherapy. *Soc Radiat Oncol Thai.*, 1998, 4(2), 22-24.

[6]   Pairatchvet, V; Narkwong, L; Puataweepong, P. High-dose-rate interstitial brachytherapy in the management of carcinoma of the uterine cervix and other gynecologic malignancies. *J Med Assoc Thai.*, 2005, 88(8), 1045-1050.

[7]   Seenukhroah, A. Verification of absorbed dose in muscle values calculated by the brachyvision software for the treatment planning of carcinoma of cervix using iridium-192 intracavitary insertion technique in Maharat Nakhon Ratchasima Hospital. *Maharat Nakhon Ratchasima Hosp Med Bull*, 2006, 30(2 Suppl), 61-66.

[8]   Peesee, M; Reamsiri, T; Khwakong, K; Ngamnaseow, N; Tungsubutra, K; Kirdpon, W. Low dose rate brachytherapy caesium-137 afterloading in the treatment of carcinoma of uterine cervix in Srinagarind Hospital: *Analysis of acturial survival rate. ASEAN J Radiol*, 1995, 1(2), 125-130.

[9]   Lorvidhaya, V; Tonusin, A; Changwiwit, W; Chitapanarux, I; Wanwilairat, S; Chawapun, N; Sukthomya, V; Srisomboon, J. High-dose-rate afterloading brachytherapy in carcinoma of the cervix : an experience of 1992 patients (24th annual scientific meeting on Mahidol' day). *Chiang Mai Med Bull.*, 2000, 39(3Suppl): 21.

[10] Pattaranutaporn, P. Iridium-192 wax mould theraphy for the treatment of superfical tumor of the floor of mouth. *ASEAN J Radiol*, 1995, 1(3), 135-139.

[11] Patjanasoontorn, B; Pesi, M; Krusun, S; Reamsiri, T; Phanmanee, A. Hign-dose-rate endobronchial brachytherapy for the locul control of intraluminal bronchogenic carcinoma (Annual Academic Convention 1998 Faculty of Medicine, Khon Kaen University. *Srinagarind Med J*, 1998, 13 9Suppl), 144.

[12] Panichevaluk, A; Prateepasen, P; Kongthanarat, Y; Sirisuk, P; Sahachjesadakul, P.Intracavitary HDR 60 Brachytherapy in the nasopharyngeal cancer patients at Rajavithi Hospital. *J Rajvithi Hosp*, 1999, 10(3), 33-39.

In: Brachytherapy
Editor: Leoni M. Fischer

ISBN: 978-1-61728-750-3
© 2011 Nova Science Publishers, Inc.

Chapter 8

Nanobrachytherapy

Viroj Wiwanitkit
Wiwanikit House, Bangkhae, Bangkok, Thailand

Abstract

Nanomedicine has become the new emerging medical science. It can be applied to many branches of medicine. Application of nanomedicineto cancer therapy can be seen, and nanobrachytherapy is the newest approach forbrachytherapy. This article will briefly discuss this new approach of brachytherapy.

What Is Nanomedicine? [1 – 3]

Nanoscience is the newest branch of science. This specific science focuses on nanomaterials, their properties and applications. The term "nano" means very small. This is not visible by the naked eye. In the nanoscale, there are several important properties of materials that change from the larger scale. These basic nanomaterials' properties are the basic things that are useful in several adaptations of nanomaterials. For example, the nanomaterial usually has electrical charge and binding properties. The accumulation of nanomaterials due to charge and binding properties can result in a larger molecule. It is not a surprise if there is only a larger molecule as an outcome. But the interesting point is the change of color that can be detected in the case of accumulation of nanomaterials.

Several branches of nanoscience have emerged in the past few years. Nanomedicine is a specific branch of nanoscience in medicine. The pathophysiology, diagnosis, treatment and prevention in nanoscale are covered by nanomedicine. At present, the drift of medical practice from macroscale and microscale can be seen and this is an exact development in medicine. At present, several areas of medical science have found their way to the nanoscale. Nanosurgery, nanodentistry, nanodiagnosis and nanotherapy are good examples. With the advent of nanomedicine, the diagnosis and treatment of previously problematic diseases can be expected. This can be the hope in medicine.

Nanooncology: Nanomedicine for Cancer[4 – 7]

As already noted, there are many focuses of nanomedicine. Nanooncology is the special focus of nanomedicine on cancer. The application of nanoscience in oncology is the new thing. With use of nanomaterials, new diagnostic tools can be developed and used for diagnosis of a malignancy. The new tools become helpful in shortening turnaround and making the diagnostic process easier. In addition, the nanoimaging technique can be applied for visualization of a tumor cell. This is very useful for detection of the tumor in an occulted area. Also, the nanodevice can be a useful approach for a deep tumor. Finally, many new drugs by nanopharmacology principles are under development and trial and have become the new hope in cancer treatment.

Focusing on cancer treatment, nanosurgery and nanopharmacology have become the main new approaches in nanooncology. Nanobrachytherapy is another way of cancer treatment that is based on nanomedicine. This technique for cancer therapy is very new and is not widely recognized. In this specific article, the author will discussthis cancer therapy technique. By name, nanobrachytherapy is a brachytherapybased on a nanomedical approach. The application of a nanomedical approach can be the use of nanomaterials as an attachment to the classical brachytherapy.

Nanobrachytherapy: What and How

As already noted, the nanobrachytherapy is the new technique of brachytherapy making use of nanomedine. This is the newest technique for brachytherapy. The real usages in human beings are not accepted at present. However, there are many reports on trials of nanobachytherapy in animal models. The important reports will be summarized and presented in Table 1.

According to Table 1, it can be seen that nanobrachytherapy still used the core concept of brachytherapy. The actual function of nanonmedical principle in nanobrachytherapy is the use of nanomaterials as an attachment to improve the classical system.

The future of nanobrachytherapy is the big query at present. Since there are still very limited reports on nanobrachytherapy, further research studies on this area are required before introduction of nanobrachytherapy for real medical practice in human beings. The control of use as well as the control of the system is necessary. Setting of a forum to increase the collaboration among medical scientists who are interested in nanobrachytherapy is recommended.

Table 1. Important reports on nanobrachytherapy

Authors	Details
Day et al. [8]	Day et al. discussed the concept of using nanoparticles This concept is the fundamental principle for nanobrachytherapy [8].
Jain [9]	Jain discusses the recent advanced nanotechnology for cancer therapy including application in photodynamics treatment [9].
Khan et al. [10]	Khan et al. first reported on fabrication of {198Au0} radioactive composite nanodevices and their use for nanobrachytherapy [10]. In this work, radioactive composite nanodevices (CND) were used as a key tool [10]. Khan et al. found that "A single intratumoral injection of poly{198Au0}(d=22nm) CNDs in phosphate-buffered saline delivering a dose of 74 muCi resulted after 8 days in a statistically significant 45% reduction in tumor volume, when compared with untreated groups and those injected with the "cold" nanodevice [10]." According to this work, there is no complication and side effect of nanoparticles. As a result, Khan et al. proposed that "This study provides the first proof of principle that radioactive CNDs can deliver therapeutic doses to tumors [10]."
Majoros et al. [11]	Majoros et al. reported on synthesis of poly(amidoamine) dendrimer-based multifunctional engineered nanodevice for cancer therapy [11]. This particle can be expected for application in nanobrachytherapy.
Majoros et al [12]	Majoros et al. reported on new alternative synthesis of poly(amidoamine) dendrimer-based multifunctional engineered nanodevice for cancer therapy [12]. In this work, the synthesized multifunctional dendrimer conjugates were tested in vitro for targeted delivery of chemotherapeutic and imaging agents to specific cancer cells and acceptable results were derived [12]. This particle can also be expected for application in nanobrachytherapy.

References

[1]   Moghimi, SM; Hunter, AC; Murray, JC. Nanomedicine: current status and future prospects.*FASEBJ*, 2005, Mar, 19(3), 311-30.

[2]   Emerich, DF. Nanomedicine--prospective therapeutic and diagnostic applications. *Expert Opin Biol Ther.*, 2005, Jan, 5(1), 1-5.

[3]   Emerich, DF; Thanos, CG. Nanotechnology and medicine.*Expert Opin Biol Ther.*, 2003, Jul, 3(4), 655-63.

[4]   Bharali, DJ; Khalil, M; Gurbuz, M; Simone, TM; Mousa, SA. Nanoparticles and cancer*Int J Nanomedicine.*, 2009, 4, 1-7.

[5]   LaRocque, J; Bharali, DJ; Mousa, SA. Cancer detection*Mol Biotechnol.*, 2009, Jul, 42(3), 358-66.

[6]   Peer, D; Karp, JM; Hong, S; Farokhzad, OC; Margalit, R; Langer, R. Nanocarriers as an emerging platform*Nat Nanotechnol*, 2007 Dec, 2(12), 751-60.

[7]   Sumer, B; Gao, J. Theranostic nanomedicine*Nanomed*, 2008 Apr, 3(2), 137-40.

[8]   Day, ES; Morton, JG; West, JL. Nanoparticles for thermal cancer.*J Biomech Eng.*, 2009, Jul, 131(7), 074001.

[9]   Jain, KK. Recent advances in nanooncology.*Technol Cancer Res Treat*, 2008, Feb, 7(1), 1-13.

[10]   Khan, MK; Minc, LD; Nigavekar, SS; Kariapper, MS; Nair, BM; Schipper, M; Cook, AC; Lesniak, WG; Balogh, LP. Fabrication of {198Au0} radioactive composite nanodevices and their use for nanobrachytherapy. *Nanomedicine.* 2008, Mar, 4(1), 57-69.

[11]   Majoros, IJ; Thomas, TP; Mehta, CB; Baker, JR; Jr. Poly(amidoamine) dendrimer-based multifunctional engineered nanodevice for cancer therapy. *J Med Chem.* 2005, Sep 22, 48(19), 5892-9.

[12]   Majoros, IJ; Myc, A; Thomas, T; Mehta, CB; Baker, JR; Jr. PAMAM dendrimer-based multifunctional conjugate for cancer therapy: synthesis, characterization, and functionality. *Biomacromolecules.* 2006, Feb, 7(2), 572-9.

In: Brachytherapy
Editor: Leoni M. Fischer

ISBN: 978-1-61728-750-3
© 2011 Nova Science Publishers, Inc.

Chapter 9

Brachytherapy for Soft Tissue Sarcomas

***Tadahiko Kubo**[*1], **Takashi Sugita**[2], **Shoji Shimose**[1],*
***Toshihiro Matsuo**[1], **Hiroaki Kimura**[3],*
***Masahiro Kenjo**[4] **and Mitsuo Ochi**[1]*

[1] Departments of Orthopaedic Surgery, Graduate Schoolof Biomedical Sciences,
Hiroshima University, 1-2-3 Kasumi,
Minami-ku, Hiroshima, 734-8551, Japan
[2] Department of Orthopaedic Surgery, Hiroshima Prefecture Hospital,
1-5-54 Ujinakanda, Minami-ku, Hiroshima, 734-8530, Japan
[3] Department of Rehabilitation, Hiroshima University Hospital,
1-2-3 Kasumi, Minami-ku, Hiroshima, 734-8551, Japan
[4] Departments of Radiology, Graduate School of Biomedical Sciences, Hiroshima
University, 1-2-3 Kasumi, Minami-ku,
Hiroshima, 734-8551, Japan

Abstract

Introduction

Limb-sparing surgery and adjuvant radiation have replaced amputation as the mainstay treatment for patients with soft tissue sarcoma (STS) of the extremity, since adjuvant radiotherapy has been shown to improve local control and disease-specific mortality. Additional brachytherapy, interstitial tumor bed irradiation, following conservative surgery represents a means of enhancing the therapeutic ratio, as biological and dosimetric advantage over external beam radiotherapy (EBRT).

* Correspondence: e-mail: kubot@hiroshima-u.ac.jp, Dr T. Kubo; telephone: 81-82-257-5232; fax: 81-82-257-5234.

Success in the management of STS is often limited by the extension of lesions to neurovascular structures. In an effort to preserve limbs, conservative surgery with adjuvant high-dose-rate (HDR) brachytherapy has been reported, whereas little is known about the tolerance of peripheral nerves to brachytherapy. The purpose of this study was to determine the oncological outcome in patients with STS treated with adjuvant HDR brachytherapy and to evaluate the efficacy and radiation neurotoxicity of HDR brachytherapy in patients with STSin contact with neurovascular bundles.

Methods

Between 1995 and 2000, 28 patients with 29 STS of the extremity and superficial trunk were treated in our institute with limb salvage surgery followed by fractionated HDR brachytherapy. Seven of the 28 cases involved theneurovascular bundle. Afterloading catheters placed within the tumor bed directly upon the preserved neurovascular structures were postoperatively loaded with Iridium-192 with a total dose of 50 Gy. To further investigate the subclinical nerve damage by HDR brachytherapy, motor nerve conduction velocity studies were carried out in 3 patients.

Results

There was one local recurrence and 8 lung metastases. Eighteen patients survived and continued to be disease-free. One patient died of heart problems. With a median follow-up period of 34 months, the 5-year actuarial overall survival and disease-free survival rates were 68.1 and 51.9%, respectively. Complications included 4 wound complications, 2 nerve damage, and one bone fracture. But there was no practical and electrophysiological finding of neurotoxicity due to HDR brachytherapy.

Discussion

This study demonstrated that conservative surgery combined with adjuvant HDR brachytherapy is the treatment of choice for patients with STS to avoid amputation or major limb function loss. Several large clinical studies have established the efficacy of conventional low-dose-rate brachytherapy as an adjuvant therapy for STS. The use of HDR is considered to be an attractive alternative, because this technique allows treatment to be given in minutes instead of days. Here, we discuss the effectiveness and complications of brachytherapy in STS, with a review of the pertinent literature.

Introduction

Soft tissue sarcomas (STS) are a relatively uncommon disease accounting for approximately 1% of all adult malignancies and 15% of pediatric malignancies [1]. They are of mesenchymal origin and may occur within any organ or at any anatomic location. There are more than 50 subtypes of soft tissue sarcoma according to their different origins and histologies [2]. The most common are malignant fibrous histiocytoma (28%), leiomyosarcoma (12%), liposarcoma (15%), synovial sarcoma (10%), and malignant peripheral nerve sheath tumours (6%) [3]. In general, STS have high potential for local recurrence (10-30%) [4-6] and distant metastases (30-45%) [7-9], despite integral multimodality therapy consisted with surgery, chemotherapy, and radiotherapy [10]. In the current context of organ and function preservation, limb-sparing surgery and adjuvant radiation have replaced amputation as the mainstay treatment for patients with STS of the extremity, since adjuvant radiotherapy has been shown to improve local control and disease-specific mortality [11-13]. Additional brachytherapy, interstitial tumor bed irradiation, following conservative surgery represents a means of enhancing the therapeutic ratio, as a biological and dosimetric advantage over external beam radiotherapy (EBRT).

Success in the management of STS is often limited by the extension of lesions to neurovascular structures, because of the difficulty in dissecting the neurovascular bundle from the tumor without compromising the function and local recurrence of residual lesions. Patients with STS involving or extending to neurovascular structures may be sometimes advised to undergo an amputation. In an effort to preserve limbs, conservative surgery with various modalitiessuch as nerve resection with or without nerve grafts, irradiation, and hyperthermia for preservation of peripheral nerves has been reported [14-17]. Brachytherapy has been shown to provide excellent local control and limb preservation in patients with STS, whereas little is known about the tolerance of peripheral nerves to brachytherapy. The placement of afterloading catheters directly upon neurovascular structures to irradiate such lesions, appropriately subjects them to a high dose of radiation. The American Brachytherapy Society suggested that brachytherapy, especially high-dose-rate (HDR) brachytherapy, should be used with caution in such situations [18].We treated 7 patients with conservative surgical resection and placement of afterloading catheters directly upon these critical structures followed by fractionated HDR brachytherapy.

The purpose of this study was to determine the oncological outcome in patients with STS treated with adjuvant HDR brachytherapy and to evaluate the efficacy and radiation neurotoxicity of HDR brachytherapy in patients with STSin contact with neurovascular bundles. Furthermore, we discuss the effectiveness and complications of brachytherapy in STS, with a review of the pertinent literature.

Materials and Methods

Patients

Between 1995 and 2000, 28 patients with 29 STS of the extremity and superficial trunk were treated in our institute with limb salvage surgery followed by fractionated HDR brachytherapy, after obtaining informed consent from the patients or their guardians. The median age at the time of the surgery was 62 years (range: 14-86). There were 18 males and 10 females. Twenty-four patients presented with a primary lesion without distant metastasis. Four patients were referred for recurrent tumors. Fourteen patients had a malignant fibrous histiocytoma, 4 patients had a liposarcoma, 2 patients had a malignant schwannoma, 2 had an extraskeletal osteosarcoma, and 6 had various histological subtypes. The tumor sites were 17 in the thigh, 5 in the forearm, 2 in the buttock, and 5 elsewhere. Five tumors were treated with wide excision, 22 tumors with marginal excision, and 2 tumors with intralesional excision. The clinical and pathological characteristics of patients and tumors are listed in Table 1.

Table 1.Patient characteristics

Features	No. of cases (%) n = 28
Age (years) Range Median ± SD	14-86 62.1± 19.8
Sex Male Female	18 (64.3) 10 (35.7)
Follow up (months) Range Median ± SD	8-81 34.2± 19.9
Site Thigh Forearm Buttock Other	17 (58.6) 5 (17.2) 2 (6.9) 5 (17.2)
Histology Malignant fibrous histiocytoma Liposarcoma Malignant schwannoma Extraskeletal osteosarcoma Other	15 (51.7) 4 (13.8) 2 (6.9) 2 (6.9) 6 (20.7)
Excision Wide Marginal Intralesional	5 (17.2) 22 (75.9) 2 (6.9)

Surgery and HDR Brachytherapy

Seven of the 28 cases involved the neurovascular bundle. All of the STS involving or adjacent to neurovascular structures could be marginally resected with careful dissection of these critical structures. The pathological examination of surgical specimens demonstrated that there were no gross residual lesions and one microscopic positive margin, which was defined as tumor cells present at the resection margins. A microscopically negative margin was defined as no tumor cells at the margins. In all of the 6 lesions with negative margins, tumor cells were seen within 1 mm from the margins at the neurovascular bundle.

The brachytherapy technique has been previously described [18,19]. In brief, the technique of brachytherapy used afterloading catheters placed intraoperatively in the tumor bed as a single plane implant. The afterloading catheters with a 1 cm spacing in between were placed within the surgical bed directly upon the preserved neurovascular bundles. The catheters were located either parallel or vertical to the limb axes. The afterloading catheters were fixed in position in the target region using absorbable sutures and secured to the skin at the catheter exit site with buttons. Postoperative localization films, along with opaque dummy sources inserted into each individual catheter, were taken to confirm the position of the catheters and for contouring and HDR brachytherapy planning. Three-dimensional treatment planning was performed by the Nucletron PLATO planning station (Nucletron Corp., Columbia, MD) according to the International Commission on Radiation Units and Measurements (ICRU) Repost 58 [20]. The clinical target volume (CTV) was defined by expanding the resected tumor bed by 0.5 cm margins. The planning target volume (PTV) was defined by expanding the CTV by1.0 cm margins on the catheter plane. Multiple dose prescription points (5 mm from the source axis) were defined in accordance with each dwell position. The prescribed dose at the periphery of the PTV was 5 Gy per fraction. The PTV was expected to cover the whole dissected portion of the nerve because the width of the nerve was less than 5 mm in all patients. Seven to ten days after the implantation, the catheters were loaded with nominal 370 GBq Iridium-192 using Microselectron-HDR (Nucletron Corp., Columbia, MD). The total dose was 50 Gy, administered as 5 Gy per fraction. Treatments were given twice a day over 5 days with a minimum of 6 hours between fractions. One patient with low-grade extraskeletal chondrosarcomaout of 29 STSreceived 30 Gy of HDR brachytherapy as a boost, combined with 20 Gy of adjuvant EBRT.

Electrophysiological Study

Motor nerve conduction velocity (MCV) of peripheral nerves was measured by standardized techniques using Nicolet VikingQuest (Nicolet Biomedical Inc., Madison, WI) at the latest follow-up. In brief, for MCV of the median nerve, supramaximal stimuli were applied to the elbow, and the compound muscle action potential was recorded from surface electrodes placed over the abductor pollicis brevis muscle. To evaluate the MCV of the sciatic nerve, F-wave conduction velocity (FWCV) of the tibial nerve was used, according to Kimura et al [21]. F responses were recorded with surface electrodes over the abductor hallucis, following supramaximal stimulation at the ankle. A total of 16 F-waves were recorded and minimal F-wave latency was determined.

Follow-up and Statistical Analysis

The time of follow-up was calculated from the date of the operation. All survival analyses were evaluated with the Kaplan-Meier product-limit method. The median follow-up period was 34 months (range: 8-81 months).

Results

Oncological Outcomes

There was one local recurrence (3.4%) and 8 lungmetastases (26.7%). The patient developed a local recurrence outside the PTVof brachytherapy 25 months postoperatively

(Figure 1). This failure was successfully salvaged with complete resection of the recurrent lesion and 50 Gy of adjuvant EBRT, but the patient experienced a femoral shaft fracture 32 months later. Eighteen patients survived and continued to be disease-free (46.3%). One patient died of heart problems. With a median follow-up period of 34 months, the 5-year actuarial overall survival and disease-free survival rates were 68.1 and 51.9%, respectively (Figure 2).

Complications

Complications included 4 delayed wound healing (13.3%, two requiring additional surgery; muscle transfer, pedicles skin flap) and one bone fracture (3.4%).

Two patients had nerve-associated complications at the time of follow-up.One patient developed an immediate postoperative palsy of the anterior interosseous nerve prior to brachytherapy. The other patient had experienced sensory loss of the tibial nerve since before treatment, possibly caused by the lesion compressing the tibial nerve. In both cases, these complications have been improving. Therefore, there was no practical evidence of HDR brachytherapy-induced neurotoxicity.

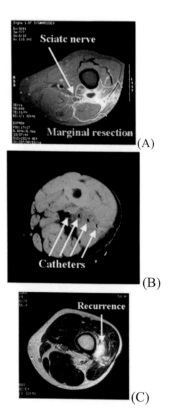

Figure 1. (A) MRI showing surgical plan for treatment of malignant fibrous histiocytoma in the thigh. (B) Postoperative CT scan showing four afterloading catheters for brachytherapy placed in surgical bed. (C) MRI taken 25 months postoperatively showing a local recurrence outside the planning target volumeof brachytherapy.

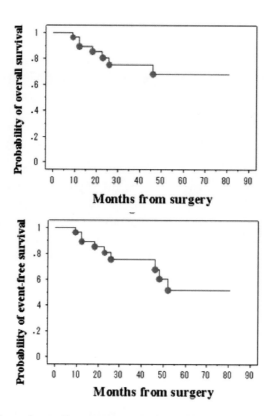

Figure. 2.Kaplan-Meier plots of overall survival (a)and disease-free survival (b) in all 28 patients with soft tissue sarcomas.

To further investigate the subclinical nerve damage by HDR brachytherapy, MCV studies were carried out. Of five survivors, two patients who had radiation-unrelated neuropathy were excluded. The MCV value of the median nerve (55.0 m/s) and FWCV values of the tibial nerves (for MCV of the sciatic nerves) (50.3, 58.5 m/s) were in the normal range [21, 22], consistent with our clinical findings.

Discussion

Brachytherapy (brachy meaning short in classic Greek) is a radiation technique in which radioisotopes are placed inside or at a short distance from the tumor. The radioisotopes most often used are cesium-137, iridium-192, and iodine-125. For urological or gynaecological cancers, radioactive sources are placed inside body cavities (intracavitary), whereas for soft tissue sarcomas radioactive material is placed directly through the tissues (interstitial). Radioactive sources can be administered during a surgical procedure alone (intraoperative), withdrawn after a specified dose has been delivered (perioperative) or left to decay inside the body (permanent). Brachytherapy can also be classified according to the prescribed dose rate as high-dose-rate (>12 Gy/h), or low-dose-rate (0.4-2 Gy/h).

The target volume definitions are based upon the ICRU report 58, Dose and Volume Specification for Reporting Interstitial Therapy [20]. The PTV refers to the volume of tissue that needs to be irradiated to ensure that the target receives the prescribed dose; the CTV is the tissue volume presumed to contain microscopic disease at a specific probability level; and the irradiated volume refers to the volume of tissue that receives a dose of radiotherapy meant to be biologically relevant because of the inaccuracies of the radiation techniques.

Oncological Outcomes

This study demonstrated that conservative surgery combined with adjuvant HDR brachytherapy is the treatment of choice for patients with STS to avoid amputation or major limb function loss. Brachytherapy has many theoretical and practical advantages, compared to EBRT. The shorter overall treatment time offers the patient conveniences and reduces the financial cost of treatment [23], in contrast to the standard 7-8 week course of EBRT. The rapid dose fall-off of brachytherapy spares more surrounding normal tissues [18].

Several large clinicalstudies have demonstrated the efficacy of conventional low-dose-rate (LDR) brachytherapy as an adjuvant therapy for STS. LDR brachytherapy provided adequate local control and acceptable morbidity compared favourably with those of EBRT [24, 25]. According to prospective randomised trials, adjuvant brachytherapy improves local control after complete resection of STS. This improvement is limited to patients with high-grade histopathology [19, 26]. Following these reports, we have been treating only high-grade STS with adjuvant brachytherapy since 1996. In this study, Patient 5 with a low-grade lesion received adjuvant brachytherapy in 1995.

Compared to LDR brachytherapy, the use of HDR is an attractive alternative, because this technique allows treatment to be given in minutes instead of days, eliminating the radiation hazards and prolonged hospital stays associated with LDR. HDR brachytherapy is expected to replace traditional LDR brachytherapy, although there is limited experience in the use of HDR, both in terms of the duration and the number of cases, compared to LDR [27, 28]. Further clinical data are needed to determine the specific role of HDR in the management of STS.

Morbidity

Wound complication has been widely evaluated as the most probable morbidity of brachytherapy (8-38%) [29-33]. In this study, 4 cases of delayed wound healing (13.3%) occurred, which is in line with other publications. Alektiar et al. conducted a large randomised trial of LDR brachytherapy versus no further radiotherapy after complete excision of 164 STS. In terms of wound complications, there is no statistical difference between the brachytherapy arm and the no-brachytherapy arm (24% vs. 14%; $P = 0.13$) [24]. Pohar et al. retrospectively analysed outcomes of patients treated with LDR versus HDR adjuvant brachytherapy as a boost of EBRT in 37 patients with STS. They reported no significant difference regarding the rate of National Cancer Institute grades 2-4 wound-healing complications (40% in the LDR vs. 18% in the HDR; $P = 0.14$) [34].

The effect of adjuvant radiation on the development of bony fractures has been reported in the literature, but the data are scant. Alectiar et al. showed an overall rate of 2% (4% in the brachytherapy vs. 0% in the no-brachytherapy;$P = 0.20$) [24]. Patients with extremity lesions who underwent bone resection and/or periosteal stripping had a significantly higher rate of bone fracture compared with those with intact bone [24, 35].

Two articles have described the direct effect of LDR brachytherapy on peripheral nerves thus far. Zelefsky et al. reported that none of the 38 patients with STS involving theneurovascular bundle developed radiation neuropathy after receiving conservative tumor resection and cumulative doses less than 9,000 cGy of LDR brachytherapy combined with or without EBRT [36]. Llaceret al. stated that 8 out of 98 patients treated with LDRintraoperativebrachytherapy had peripheral neuropathy and fibrosis. But they did not find any significant risk factors for developing neuropathy, maybe because of the low occurrence [37]. A histological and electrophysiological study using rabbits observed good tolerance of irradiation by iridium-192 LDR brachytherapy of doses up to 13,000 cGy on the carotid-sheath contents including the vagus nerve [38].

There are no clinical reports which properly evaluate HDR brachytherapy-inducing neuropathy, and no experimental studies on nerve tolerance to HDR brachytherapy. In general, HDR brachytherapy is believed to carry a large risk of nerve damage. It has been proposed that a layer of gel-foam or muscle should be interposed between the catheters and the neurovascular bundles [39, 40]. Nevertheless, the results of our study showed that there was no practical and electrophysiological finding of neurotoxicity of HDR brachytherapy. Based on their clinical study [36], Zelefsky et al. speculated that the threshold tolerance of peripheral nerves to LDR brachytherapy might be higher than to EBRT.Similarly, HDR brachytherapy may have a higher threshold tolerance than EBRT, attributable to different radioactive sources.

Despite the small number of patients, our findings suggest that HDR brachytherapy may not adversely affect peripheral nerve function in the treatment of STS with neurovascular involvement. Latency also needs to be considered in evaluation of radiation neuropathy. A long-term follow-up study of EBRT reported that the incidence of complications involving nerves increased with time after radiation and not all of the cases were detected at 5, or even 10 years after the treatment [41]. More clinical data with a large number of patients treated with HDR brachytherapy and longer follow-up periods are required to detect further long-term morbidity.

Recent Developments

The pulse dose-rate (PDR) brachytherapy is a new modality that combines the undisputed physical advantages of HDR technology (isodose optimisation and radiation safety) with the radiobiological advantages of LDR. Lazzaro et al. reported that PDR interstitial brachytherapy for STS is an effective, well-tolerated adjuvant radiation treatment that offers several practical advantages such as low toxicity, overall shorter radiotherapy, and reduced hospitalisation [42].

The recent dramatic advances in technology have impacted on the practice of brachytherapy in 2 main areas: treatment delivery, such as customised templates for the applicator setting and flab applicators [43, 44], and treatment planning. Until recently, brachytherapy planning and dosimetry were based on fixed rules and fixed sources according to the traditional schools of Manchester dosimetry and the Paris rules for interstitial therapy [45]. Often, however, they could not be fulfilled completely and even the most experienced brachytherapist will not always achieve a perfect implant with consequent adverse effects on dosimetry. These fixed rules have been replaced by computer-assisted dose calculations around a brachytherapy implant [46, 47] and 3-dimensional image-based treatment-planning systems [48-51].

Conclusion

This study demonstrated that conservative surgery combined with adjuvant HDR brachytherapy is the treatment of choice for patients with STS to avoid amputation or major limb function loss. Our findings also suggested that HDR brachytherapy might not adversely affect nerve function in the treatment of STS with neurovascular involvement. Despite the small number of patients, our encouraging results are valuable for limb-preserving surgery of unmanageable STSinvolving critical neurovascular structures.

References

[1]   Greenlee, R. T., Murray, T., Bolden, S. & Wingo, P. A. (2000). Cancer statistics, 2000. *CA Cancer J Clin.*, *50*, 7-33.

[2]   Enzinger, F. M. & Weiss, S. W. (1995). Soft tissue tumors. 3rd. St. *Louis*, Missouri: Mosby.

[3]   Coindre, J. M., Terrier, P., Guillou, L., Le Doussal, V., Collin, F., Ranchere, D., Sastre, X., Vilain, M. O.., Bonichon, F. & N'Guyen Bui, B. (2001). Predictive value of grade for metastasis development in the main histologic types of adult soft tissue sarcomas: a study of 1240 patients from the French Federation of Cancer Centers Sarcoma Group. *Cancer*, *91*, 1914-1926.

[4]   Lindberg, R. D., Martin, R. G., Romsdahl, M. M. & Barkley, H. T., Jr. (1981). Conservative surgery and postoperative radiotherapy in 300 adults with soft-tissue sarcomas. *Cancer*, *47*, 2391-2397.

[5]   Potter, D. A., Kinsella, T., Glatstein, E., Wesley, R., White, D. E., Seipp, C. A., Chang, A. E., Lack, E. E., Costa, J. & Rosenberg, S. A. (1986). High-grade soft tissue sarcomas of the extremities. *Cancer*, *58*, 190-205.

[6]   Rooser, B., Berg, N. O., Ranstam, J., Rydholm, A. & Willen, H. (1990). Prediction of survival in patients with high-grade soft tissue sarcoma. *Int Orthop*, *14*, 199-204.

[7]   Collin, C., Godbold, J., Hajdu, S. & Brennan, M. (1987). Localized extremity soft tissue sarcoma: an analysis of factors affecting survival. *J Clin Oncol*, *5*, 601-612.

[8]   Pisters, P. W., Leung, D. H., Woodruff, J., Shi, W. & Brennan, M. F. (1996). Analysis of prognostic factors in 1,041 patients with localized soft tissue sarcomas of the extremities.*J Clin Oncol*, *14*, 1679-1689.

[9]   Ruka, W., Emrich, L. J., Driscoll, D. L. & Karakousis, C. P. (1988). Prognostic significance of lymph node metastasis and bone, major vessel, or nerve involvement in adults with high-grade soft tissue sarcomas. *Cancer*, *62*, 999-1006.

[10] Pitcher, M. E., Fish, S. & Thomas, J. M. (1994). Management of soft tissue sarcoma. *Br J Surg., 81*, 1136-1139.

[11] Rosenberg, S. A., Tepper, J., Glatstein, E., Costa, J., Young, R., Baker, A., Brennan, M. F., Demoss, E. V., Seipp, C., Sindelar, W. F., Sugarbaker, P. & Wesley, R.(1983). Prospective randomized evaluation of adjuvant chemotherapy in adults with soft tissue sarcomas of the extremities. *Cancer, 52*, 424-434.

[12] Williard, W. C., Hajdu, S. I., Casper, E. S. & Brennan, M. F. (1992). Comparison of amputation with limb-sparing operations for adult soft tissue sarcoma of the extremity. *Ann Surg., 215*, 269-275.

[13] Yang, J. C., Chang, A. E., Baker, A. R., Sindelar, W. F., Danforth, D. N., Topalian, S. L., DeLaney, T., Glatstein, E., Steinberg, S. M., Merino, M. J. & Rosenberg, S. A. (1998). Randomized prospective study of the benefit of adjuvant radiation therapy in the treatment of soft tissue sarcomas of the extremity. *J Clin Oncol, 16*, 197-203.

[14] Kawai, A., Miyakawa, T., Senda, M., Endo, H., Naito, N., Umeda, M. & Inoue, H. (2002). Gait characteristics after limb-sparing surgery with sciatic nerve resection: a report of two cases. *J Bone Joint Surg Am., 84*, 264-268.

[15] Koshima, I., Nanba, Y., Tsutsui, T., Takahashi, Y. & Kawai, A. (2003). Vascularized femoral nerve graft with anterolateral thigh true perforator flap for massive defects after cancer ablation in the upper arm. *J Reconstr Microsurg, 19*, 299-302.

[16] Gillette, E. L., Mahler, P. A., Powers, B. E., Gillette, S. M. & Vujaskovic, Z. (1995). Late radiation injury to muscle and peripheral nerves. *Int J Radiat Oncol Biol Phys., 31*, 1309-1318.

[17] Emami, B., Scott, C., Perez, C. A., Asbell, S., Swift, P., Grigsby, P., Montesano, A., Rubin, P., Curran, W., Delrowe, J., Arastu, H., Fu, K. & Moros, E. (1996). Phase III study of interstitial thermoradiotherapy compared with interstitial radiotherapy alone in the treatment of recurrent or persistent human tumors. A prospectively controlled randomized study by the Radiation Therapy Group. *Int J Radiat Oncol Biol Phys., 34*, 1097-1104.

[18] Nag, S., Shasha, D., Janjan, N., Petersen, I. & Zaider, M. (2001). The American Brachytherapy Society recommendations for brachytherapy of soft tissue sarcomas. *Int J Radiat Oncol Biol Phys., 49*, 1033-1043.

[19] Pisters, P. W., Harrison, L. B., Woodruff, J. M., Gaynor, J. J. & Brennan, M. F. (1994).A prospective randomized trial of adjuvant brachytherapy in the management of low-grade soft tissue sarcomas of the extremity and superficial trunk.*J Clin Oncol,12*,1150-1155.

[20] Chassagne, D., Dutreix, A., Ash, D., Hanson, W. F., Visser, A. G. & Wilson, J. F. (1997). Dose and Volume Specification for Reporting Interstitial Therapy. ICRU Report No.58, Bethesda, Maryland: *Internal Commission on Radiation Units and Measurements.*

[21] Kimura, J., Bosch, P. & Lindsay, G. M. (1975). F-wave conduction velocity in the central segment of the peroneal and tibial nerves. *Arch Phys Med Rehabil, 56*, 492-497.

[22] Buschbacher, R. M. (1999). Median nerve motor conduction to the abductor pollicis brevis. *Am J Phys Med Rehabil.78* (Suppl 6), S1-S8.

[23] Janjan, N. A., Yasko, A. W., Reece, G. P., Miller, M. J., Murray, J. A., Ross, M. I., Romsdahl, M. M., Oswald, M. J., Ochran, T. G. & Pollock, R. E. (1994). Comparison

of charges related to radiotherapy for soft-tissue sarcomas treated by preoperative external-beam irradiation versus interstitial implantation. *Ann Surg Oncol*, *1*, 415-422.

[24] Alektiar, K. M., Zelefsky, M. J. & Brennan, M. F. (2000). Morbidity of adjuvant brachytherapy in soft tissue sarcoma of the extremity and superficial trunk. *Int J Radiat Oncol Biol Phys.*, *47*, 1273-1279.

[25] Alektiar, K. M., Leung, D., Zelefsky, M. J., Healey, J. H. & Brennan, M. F. (2002). Adjuvant brachytherapy for primary high-grade soft tissue sarcoma of the extremity. *Ann Surg Oncol*, *9*, 48-56.

[26] Pisters, P. W., Harrison, L. B., Leung, D. H., Woodruff, J. M., Casper, E. S. & Brennan, M. F. (1996). Long-term results of a prospective randomized trial of adjuvant brachytherapy in soft tissue sarcoma. *J Clin Oncol*, *14*, 859-868.

[27] Nag, S., Tippin, D. & Ruymann, F. B. (2003). Long-term morbidity in children treated with fractionated high-dose-rate brachytherapy for soft tissue sarcomas. *J Pediatr Hematol Oncol*, *25*, 448-452.

[28] Ballo, M. T. & Lee, A. K. (2003). Current results of brachytherapy for soft tissue sarcoma.*Curr Opin Oncol*, *15*, 313-318.

[29] Alekhteyar, K. M., Leung, D. H., Brennan, M. F. &Harrison, L. B. (1996). The effect of combined external beam radiotherapy and brachytherapy on local control and wound complications in patients with high-grade soft tissue sarcomas of the extremity with positive microscopic margin. *Int J Radiat Oncol Biol Phys.*, *36*, 321-324.

[30] Delannes, M., Thomas, L., Martel, P., Bonnevialle, P., Stoeckle, E., Chevreau, C., Bui, B. N., Daly-Schveitzer, N., Pigneux, J. & Kantor, G. (2000). Low-dose-rate intraoperative brachytherapy combined with external beam irradiation in the conservative treatment of soft tissue sarcoma. *Int J Radiat Oncol Biol Phys.*, *47*, 165-169.

[31] Andrews, S. F., Anderson, P. R., Eisenberg, B. L., Hanlon, A. L. &Pollack, A. (2004). Soft tissue sarcomas treated with postoperative external beam radiotherapy with and without low-dose-rate brachytherapy. *Int J Radiat Oncol Biol Phys.*, *59*, 475-480.

[32] Martinez-Monge, R., San Julian, M., Amillo, S., Cambeiro, M., Arbea, L., Valero, J., Gonzalez-Cao, M. & Martin-Algarra, S. (2005). Perioperative high-dose-rate brachytherapy in soft tissue sarcomas of the extremity and superficial trunk in adults: initial results of a pilot study.*Brachytherapy*, *4*, 264-270.

[33] Aronowitz, J. N., Pohar, S. S., Liu, L., Haq, R. & Damron, T. A. (2006). Adjuvant high dose rate brachytherapy in the management of soft tissue sarcoma: a dose-toxicity analysis. *Am J Clin Oncol*, *29*, 508-513.

[34] Pohar, S., Haq, R., Liu, L., Koniarczyk, M., Hahn, S., Damron, T. & Aronowitz, J. N. (2007). Adjuvant high-dose-rate and low-dose-rate brachytherapy with external beam radiation in soft tissue sarcoma: a comparison of outcomes. *Brachytherapy*, *6*, 53-57.

[35] Lin, P. P., Schupak, K. D., Boland, P. J., Brennan, M. F. & Healey, J. H. (1998). Pathologic femoral fracture after periosteal excision and radiation for the treatment of soft tissue sarcoma. *Cancer*, *82*, 2356-2365.

[36] Zelefsky, M J., Nori, D., Shiu, M. H. & Brennan, M. F. (1990). Limb salvage in soft tissue sarcomas involving neurovascular structures using combined surgical resection and brachytherapy.*Int J Radiat Oncol Biol Phys.*, *19*, 913-918.

[37] Llacer, C., Delannes, M., Minsat, M., Stoeckle, E., Votron, L., Martel, P., Bonnevialle, P., Nguyen Bui, B., Chevreau, C., Kantor, G., Daly-Schveitzer, N. & Thomas, L.

(2006). Low-dose intraoperative brachytherapy in soft tissue sarcomas involving neurovascular structure. *Radiother Oncol, 78*, 10-16.

[38] Werber, J. L., Sood, B., Alfieri, A., McCormick, S. A. & Vikram, B. (1991). Tolerance of the carotid-sheath contents to brachytherapy: an experimental study. *Laryngoscope, 101*, 587-591.

[39] Koizumi, M., Inoue, T., Yamazaki, H., Teshima, T., Tanaka, E., Yoshida, K., Imai, A., Shiomi, H., Kagawa, K., Araki, N., Kuratsu, S., Uchida, A. & Inoue, T. (1999). Perioperative fractionated high-dose rate brachytherapy for malignant bone and soft tissue tumors. *Int J Radiat Oncol Biol Phys., 43*, 989-993.

[40] Chun, M., Kang, S., Kim, B. S. & Oh, Y. T. (2001). High dose rate interstitial brachytherapy in soft tissue sarcoma: technical aspects and results. *Jpn J Clin Oncol, 31*, 279-283.

[41] Johansson, S., Svensson, H. & Denekamp, J. (2000). Timescale of evolution of late radiation injury after postoperative radiotherapy of breast cancer patients. *Int J Radiat Oncol Biol Phys., 48*, 745-750.

[42] Lazzaro, G., Lazzari, R., Pelosi, G., De Pas, T., Mariani, L., Mazzarol, G., Sances, D., Tosti, G., Baldini, F., Mosconi, M., Tedeschi, I., Viale, G., Marsiglia, H., Chiappa, A., Vavassori, A., Orecchia, R. & Testori, A. (2005). Pulsed dose-rate perioperative interstitial brachytherapy for soft tissue sarcomas of the extremities and skeletal muscles of the trunk. *Ann Surg Oncol, 12*, 935-942.

[43] Rachbauer, F., Sztankay, A., Kreczy, A., Sununu, T., Bach, C., Nogler, M., Krismer, M., Eichberger, P., Schiestl, B. & Lukas, P. (2003). High-dose-rate intraoperative brachytherapy (IOHDR) using flab technique in the treatment of soft tissue sarcomas. *Strahlenther Onkol, 179*, 480-485.

[44] Baumert, B. G., Infanger, M., Reiner, B. & Davis, J. B. (2004). A novel technique using customised templates for the application of fractionated interstitialHDR brachytherapy to the tumour bed in soft-tissue sarcomas located in the extremities. *Clin Oncol (R Coll Radiol), 16*, 457-460.

[45] Hoskin, P. J. & Bownes, P. (2006). Innovative technologies in radiation therapy: brachytherapy. *Semin Radiat Oncol, 16*, 209-217.

[46] Nath, R., Anderson, L. L., Luxton, G., Weaver, K. A., Williamson, J. F. & Meigooni, A. S. (1995). Dosimetry of interstitial brachytherapy sources: recommendations of the AAPM Radiation Therapy Committee Task Group No. 43. American Association of Physicists in Medicine. *Med Phys., 22*, 209-234.

[47] Rivard, M. J., Coursey, B. M., DeWerd, L. A., Hanson, W. F., Huq, M. S., Ibbott, G. S., Mitch, M. G., Nath, R. & Williamson, J. F. (2004). Update of AAPM Task Group No. 43 Report: A revised AAPM protocol for brachytherapy dose calculations. *Med Phys., 31*, 633-674.

[48] Moerland, M. A., van der Laarse, R., Luthmann, R. W., Wijrdeman, H. K. & Battermann, J. J. (2000). The combined use of the natural and the cumulative dose-volume histograms in planning and evaluation of permanent prostatic seed implants. *Radiother Oncol, 57*, 279-284.

[49] Potter, R., Haie-Meder, C., Van Limbergen, E., Barillot, I., De Brabandere, M., Dimopoulos, J., Dumas, I., Erickson, B., Lang, S., Nulens, A., Petrow, P., Rownd, J. & Kirisits, C. (2006). GEC ESTRO Working Group. Recommendations from gynaecological (GYN) GEC ESTRO working group (II): concepts and terms in 3D

image-based treatment planning in cervix cancer brachytherapy-3D dose volume parameters and aspects of 3D image-based anatomy, radiation physics, radiobiology. *Radiother Oncol*, *78*, 67-77.

[50] Potter, R., Dimopoulos, J., Georg, P., Lang, S., Waldhausl, C., Wachter-Gerstner, N., Weitmann, H., Reinthaller, A., Knocke, T. H., Wachter, S. & Kirisits, C. (2007). Clinical impact of MRI assisted dose volume adaptation and dose escalation in brachytherapy of locally advanced cervix cancer. *Radiother Oncol*, *83*, 148-155.

[51] Li, S., Frassica, D., DeWeese, T., Lee, D. J., Geng, J. & Nag, S. (2003). A real-time image-guided intraoperative high-dose-rate brachytherapy system. *Brachytherapy*, *2*, 5-16.

In: Brachytherapy
Editor: Leoni M. Fische

ISBN: 978-1-61728-750-3
© 2011 Nova Science Publishers, Inc.

Chapter 10

Metallic Selfexpandable Stents Combined with Intraluminal Brachytherapy in the Treatment of Nonresectable Biliary Malignancies

Radan Bruha[1], Jaromir Petrtyl [1], Martina Kubecova [3],
Petr Urbanek[4], Tomislav Svestka[1], Milan Kalab[1],
Simona Chocholova[2], Milena Mikova[2] and Zdenek Marecek[4]*

[1]4th Internal Clinic, General Teaching Hospital,
Charles University, Prague, Czech Republic
[2]Department of Radiology, General Teaching Hospital,
Charles University, Prague, Czech Republic
[3]Department of Radiotherapy and Oncology, General Teaching Hospital,
Charles University, Prague, Czech Republic
[4]Teaching Hospital, Prague 10, Internal Clinic,
Central Military Hospital, Prague, , Czech Republic

Abstract

Introduction

Gallbladder carcinoma has an extremely bad prognosis. The radical surgery is acceptable for minority of patients; external radiotherapy or chemotherapy is ineffective. The aim of study was to evaluate the therapeutic effect of a combination of intraluminal

---

*Mailing address: e-mail: bruha@cesnet.cz, Radan Bruha,MD. 4th Internal Clinic, General Teaching Hospital, Charles University. U nemocnice 2, 128 08 Prague 2. Czech Republic. Europe. Tel.: ++4202 2496 2506.

brachytherapy (ILBT) and metallic stent implantation in the treatment of patients with nonresectable biliary tumours.

Patients and Methods

43 patients aged 41-80 years with nonresectable biliary malignancies - gallbladder carcinoma (n=14), Klatskin´s tumour (n=25) and carcinoma of papilla Vateri (n=4) were treated with a combination of ILBT (Ir 192, high dose radiation, total dose 30 Gy) and metallic stent implantation (ELLA CS®). ILBT and stent insertion were performed through percutaneous drainage in all patients.

Results

The mean survival in patients with gallbladder carcinoma was 219 days (range 86-609, median 190 days) in patients with Klatskin´s tumour 483 days (range 85-1223, median 436 days) and in patients with carcinoma of papilla Vateri 850 days (range 48-1518, median 917 days). The rate of 2-year survival in these groups was 0%, 20% and 50% respectively. The survival time differed significantly. The mean time of stent patency was 203, 434 and 850 days respectively. No complications related directly to ILBT were observed.

Conclusion

ILBT combined with percutaneous stent implantation is a safe method and appears to prolong survival in inoperable patients with Klatskin´s tumour and carcinoma of papilla Vateri. No similar effect was observed in patients with gallbladder carcinoma.

Keywords: Gallbladder carcinoma, biliary tumours, percutaneous biliary drainage, self-expandable stent, intraluminal brachytherapy

Introduction

Primary tumours of the biliary tract represent 1-2% of the total number of malignancies in the population[18]. The treatment regimen of patients with these tumours depends on early diagnosis, localisation and spread of the tumour.

Cholangiocarcinomas arising from the common hepatic duct and the confluence of hepatic ducts, called Klatskin's tumours, are slow growing adenocarcinomas with late metastases, presenting mainly as obstructive jaundice [21]. Surgical resection is the only curative treatment [4], but at the time of diagnosis only 7-20% of these tumours are suitable for resection [39]. Derivation of the bile surgically, endoscopically or radiologically is a basic palliation, having the progression of the tumour unaffected [43]. Radiotherapy and chemotherapy have been tried for tumour mass reduction, but bile duct patency can not be achieved with these methods alone. Hence the idea of combination therapy [5].

Patients and Methods

Patients

Between September 1993 and December 2005, 43 patients with nonresectable tumours of the biliary tree were treated with intraluminal brachytherapy and subsequent metallic stent implantation: 25 with hilar carcinoma (Klatskin's tumour), 15 with gallbladder carcinoma and 4 with carcinoma of papilla Vateri. The demographic data are given in Tables 1-3.

The classification of patients with Klatskin's tumour (group A) was based on the Bismuth classification [3]. Patients in stage III and IV were age-matched. 5 patients in this group underwent surgery (explorative laparotomy without resection or surgical bypass), the rest were evaluated as nonresectable on radiologic and endoscopic examination (intrahepatic ductal extension, vascular invasion). The mean time from diagnosis to drainage was 2.3 months (0-17 months).

Table 1. Demographic data, survival time and stent patency in patients with Klatskin´s cholangiocarcinoma

Patient No	Sex	Age (years)	Klatskin class	Biopsy specimen obtained	Survival (days)	Stent pa-tency (days)
1	M	66	III	Autopsy	485	485
2	M	80	II	PTI* biopsy	546	293
3	M	68	III	Autopsy	223	223
4	M	60	III	Surgery	836	836
5	M	43	IV	Surgery	733	733
6	M	41	IV	Surgery	120	120
7	M	62	III	Autopsy	985	985
8	M	64	IV	Autopsy	161	145
9	M	54	III	PTI biopsy	1110	1001
10	F	71	IV	-	1223	1069
11	M	73	IV	ERCP brush	436	436
12	F	67	III	-	475	475
13	F	74	IV	Autopsy	85	85
14	F	66	IV	PTI biopsy	358	261
15	F	67	IV	Fine needle biopsy	403	131
16	F	41	IV	PTI biopsy	205	205
17	M	74	IV	PTI biopsy	554	554
18	F	57	III	Surgery	537	380
19	M	67	IV	Surgery	380	280
20	F	65	III	PTI biopsy	443	413
21	F	57	III	Autopsy	347	347
22	M	60	IV	Fine needle biopsy	545	518
23	F	62	III	-	421	421
24	M	65	III	Fine needle biopsy	355	355
25	M	71	IV	PTI biopsy	122	122
Mean		63			483.5	434

*PTI – Percutaneous intraluminal

While chemotherapy is not suitable for this type of cancer [11], radiotherapy was considered in combination with other methods - surgery or endoscopy [31]. Intraluminal brachytherapy in combination with of self-expandable metallic stent implantation seems to be a suitable method [46]. The intraluminal source allows a high local dose of radiation while exposure to adjacent radiosensitive organs is minimal [20]. Promising results with this combination therapy have been reported [7, 15]. A combination of local irradiation with external beam irradiation was suggested in some studies [17].

The purpose of the present study was to assess the impact of combined therapy on survival, quality of life and stent patency in patients with nonresectable tumours of the biliary tree.

All patients with gallbladder carcinoma (group B) underwent surgery, but without radical solution. The mean time from diagnosis to drainage was 2.5 (1-5) months.

Table 2. Demographic data, type of tumour, survival time and stent patency in patients with gallbladder carcinoma

Patient No	Sex	Age (years)	Biopsy specimen obtained	Survival (days)	Stent patency (days)
1	M	74	surgery	137	121
2	F	65	surgery	92	92
3	M	69	autopsy	234	234
4	M	64	surgery	176	143
5	M	68	surgery	609	609
6	F	56	surgery	210	152
7	F	58	surgery	397	397
8	F	63	surgery	189	114
9	F	63	surgery	225	225
10	F	59	surgery	192	192
11	F	61	surgery	213	173
12	M	69	surgery	127	127
13	M	64	surgery	180	180
14	F	67	surgery	86	86
Mean		64		219	203

Table 3. Demographic data, type of tumour, survival time and stent patency in patients with carcinoma of papila Vateri

Patient No	Sex	Age (years)	Biopsy specimen obtained	Survival (days)	Stent patency (days)
1	M	76	ERCP forceps biopsy	1277	1277
2	M	73	autopsy	557	557
3	M	80	ERCP forceps biopsy	1518	1518
4	M	76	ERCP forceps biopsy	48	48
Mean		76.2		850	850

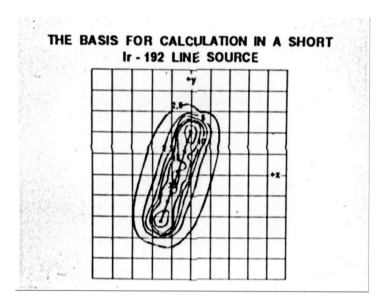

Figure 1. Calculation of isodoses for intraluminal irradiation through the external-internal drainage of biliary tree.

None of the patients with carcinoma of papilla Vateri (group C) were eligible for surgery due to concomitant disease and age. The mean time from diagnosis to drainage was 1.0 (0-2) month.

The age of patients with carcinoma of papilla Vateri was significantly higher, than in other groups.

Methods

All patients had transhepatic internal-external biliary drainage ("Wilson - COOK Medical" drainage set, diameter 9 F) (41). Intraluminal brachytherapy was performed using the automatic afterloading system Gammamed 12i (High-dose rate - HDR) with Ir ^{192} as the source. The catheter for iridium wire (diameter 5 F) was placed through the percutaneous external-internal biliary drainage catheter under fluoroscopic control. The borderline for irradiation was 1 cm distal to and 1 cm proximal to the tumour stenosis. The total dose calculated at 1 cm radius from the source was 30 Gy (Figure 1) divided into 6 sessions (5 Gy per session), each session lasting 2-8 minutes. The sessions were repeated 2 - 3 times in a week; the thin catheter for the Ir ^{192} source was removed between sessions to sustain the biliary drainage.

After the irradiation, the metallic self-expanding stents were placed percutaneously into the stenosis. Self-expandable non-covered metallic stents (ELLA, CZ – Figure 2, 3, 4, 5) were used in all patients. The stent diameter was 8-10 mm. Two stents were placed in 2 patients with Klatskin´s tumour and 1 patient with gallbladder carcinoma. Three stents were placed in 3 patients with Klatskin´s tumour (one in the left hepatic duct, another in the right hepatic duct and a 3rd one in the common hepatic duct). The remaining 37 patients had only one stent placed in for primary treatment.

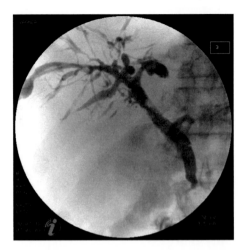

Figure 2. Percutaneous cholangiography through external drain in patient with gallbladder carcinoma showing implanted metallic stent in the upper and middle part of biliary duct.

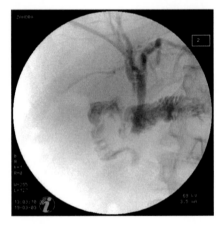

Figure 3. Percutaneous cholangiography through external drain in patient with gallbladder carcinoma showing implanted metallic stent in the upper and middle part of biliary duct.

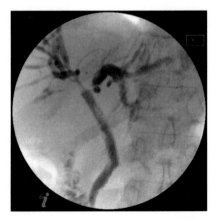

Figure 4. Percutaneous cholangiography through external drain in patient with Klatskin´s tumour III A showing metallic stent in the hepaticus communis (implanted after intraluminal irradiation).

Antibiotics were given only patients with sings of infection (fever, chills, elevated C-reactive protein, positive bacteriology). Parenteral cephalosporins or chinolones were used for initial treatment, until the chemosensitivity of infective agent was not known.

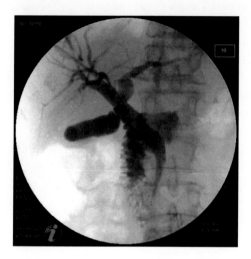

Figure 5. Percutaneous cholangiography through external drain in patient with carcinoma of papila Vateri showing implanted metallic stent in the distal part of biliary duct.

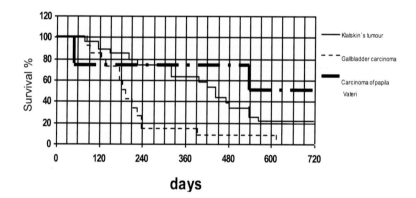

days

Figure 6. Survival of patients in different groups. Kaplan-Meier method.

Table 4. Basic statistical characteristics of survival time in different group of patients

Tumour	No of patients	Mean*	Median*	SD**	Range*	1-year survival	2-year survival
Klatskin´s	25	483	436	292	85-1223	56%	20%
Gallbladder	14	219	190	130	86-609	14%	0%
Papila of Vateri	4	850	917	582	48-1518	75%	50%

*Days, **Standard deviation in days.

External beam radiotherapy was used in two patients with Klatskin´s tumour.

Chemotherapy was used in addition to radiation in 2 patients with Klatskin´s tumour and in 2 patients with gallbladder carcinoma. All these four patients had had an arterial portcatheter, inserted into the hepatic artery during previous surgery to deliver the chemotherapeutic (5-fluorouracil and Mitomycine in all three cases) into the hepatic artery.

All patients took Ursodeoxycholic acid 750 mg p.o. daily after stent implantation to prevent bile sludge and clotting in the stent lumen.

The patients were followed up at our outpatient department at 3-month intervals. If stent occlusion was suspected, PTC or ERCP reintervention followed, except in terminal patients. In three patients, redilatation with a balloon catheter and implantation of a second metallic stent was necessary. In another two patients, a plastic endoprosthesis was implanted into the lumen of the primary metallic stent for reasons of obstruction.

Statistical methods: Mann-Whitney test (comparison of demografical data in different groups), Chi-square test (comparison of stent patency and age of patients, comparison of survival between different groups), Cox regression test (correlation of survival and age of patients), Cox-F-test (correlation of survival between different groups of patients). Survival probability curves were plotted using the Kaplan-Meier method.

Results

Data from all patients were used for follow up. Survival times calculated from the date of percutaneous drainage are given in Tables 1-4.

The survival time in different groups of patients shows significant differences (Group A versus group B at p=0.006, between all three groups at p=0.027) (Figure 6).

The mean time of stent patency was 434 days, 203 days, and 850 days in groups A, B, and C respectively. As for deceased patients with Klatskin´s tumour, 15 had no sings of stent obstruction while 10 patients had stent obstructed. In the gallbladder carcinoma group, 6 patients died with sings of stent obstruction, 8 patients with the stent patent.

In the group with carcinoma of papilla Vateri, all patients had no sings of biliary obstruction. The age had no significant influence on stent patency in any group of patients. Laboratory parameters before and after treatment are given in Table 5.

Complications: No death resulting from complications of percutaneous drainage or irradiation occurred. Pain of different intensity at the site of drainage as the most frequent complication was present in all patients. Analgetics were usually necessary for 24-48 hours after drainage.

Table 5. Mean +- SD of laboratory findings
before and two weeks after stent insertion

Tumour	Bilirubin (µmol/l)*		Alkaline phosphatase (µkat/l)**	
	Before	After	before	after
Klatskin´s	219.4±42.3	28.9±44.5	9.85±4.9	4.04±3.01
Gallbladder	183.4±161.8	26.9±17.1	7.25±4.78	6.55±4.17
Papilla of Vateri	225.8±37.4	25.8±18.8	5.79±1.62	3.35±1.08

*Normal value below 21.4 µmol/l, **normal value below 1.85 µkat/l.

Transient hemobilia was observed in 5 patients, no bleeding into the peritoneal cavity was noted. As a serious complication, there was one case of external-internal drainage displacement with bile leak into the peritoneal cavity with peritoneal irritation. In this case repeated PTC with drainage was performed, and peritonitis was treated conservatively with success.

No serious infectious complications of drainage or radiation procedure were observed. 18 patients had to be given antibiotics for bile duct infection. 1 patient developed bronchopneumonia during hospitalisation. In 2 patients transient pleural effusion appeared on the right side.

Discussion

Klatskin´s tumours are slow growing, sclerosing adenocarcinomas with dense fibroblastic reaction and circular stricture of involved ducts. Symptoms leading to diagnosis usually result from biliary stenosis - icterus, pruritus, fever, chills. Prognosis depends strongly on early diagnosis and appropriate treatment regimen. Radical resection is undoubtedly a method of choice [3]. Survival rates of 1, 2 and 5-years can be up to 66%, 32% and 8% with relatively low perioperative mortality of 2%-26% [4,39]. A distress practise of many physicians is that a patient presenting with typical symptoms is suitable for radical surgery rarely. Merits of this evidence are above all an anatomical extent of tumour - invasion of vessels, involvement of both hepatic lobes, metastases in nodules[35] followed by the patient´s condition and other accompanying diseases. It seems in this case that a surgical palliative bypass has no advantage over endoscopical or radiological methods [2]. Palliative surgery has a high postoperative mortality (up to 35%) and morbidity (up to 43%) [39,20,23] with survival times not exceeding 6 - 7 months [23].

Improvement in diagnostic methods and more precise staging of hilar tumours (including endosonography) decreased the rate of palliative surgery in patients with Klatskin´s tumour operated on at many centres only when considered fit for radical resection [47]. Inoperable cases are referred for endoscopic or radiologic methods - implantation of metallic or plastic stents percutaneously or endoscopically [14, 25].

The use of metallic stents seems to be superior to plastic endoprostheses [24]. The patency of plastic endoprosthesis (used in combination with brachytherapy) will not last longer than 3-4 months on average [13]. Exchange of an occluded internal plastic stent is possible only endoscopically; in cases of hilar stenosis, technical complication may arise, and the diameter of an endoscopical stent is much smaller than that of a stent implanted percutaneously. Another possibility is the implantation of definitive pecutaneous internal-external biliary drainage, which is easy to exchange, but the patient´s comfort is much greater with a metallic stent without external drainage. Different types of metallic stents are in use while Iridium 192 as a radiation source is used almost uniformly.

Metallic stents now represent standard palliative treatment for malignant biliary obstruction in patients with prognosis longer than a few months (not only with Klatskin´s tumours). The median patency of a metallic stent can be up to 10-12 months regardless of the stent type [8,36,26]. On the other hand, the technique of stent implantation is crucial. It is essential to place the stent far enough above and below the stenosis (overstenting) [26].

Covered stents are suitable for strictures distal to bifurcation. If implanted intrahepatically the stent cover can occlude small branches of the hepatic ducts.

If necessary we always tried to drain both the left and the right hepatic ducts in the "T" configuration. The drainage of both hepatic ducts significantly decreases the incidence of infection[14, 25]. Such complications are also prevented with large-diameter metallic stents (8-10 mm). A definitive internal metallic stent prevents also complications from the displacement of a plastic tube.

As mentioned above, the implantation of plastic or metallic stent has no influence on the growth of the tumour mass. Radiotherapy has been tried in the form of external beam radiotherapy [16], intraluminal brachytherapy over percutaneous [6, 12], ERCP [38], perioperatively inserted catheter or perioperative interstitial therapy [9].

We used the percutaneous access to the biliary tree, because endoscopic implantation of stents into the stenosis localized in liver hilum or intrahepatically is complicated and often unsuccessful. Moreover, intraluminal irradiation is easier to perform through a percutaneous catheter.

There are a number of studies using intraluminal brachytherapy and stent implantation for the treatment of patients with biliary tree malignancies. Comparison is difficult because the selection of patients, treatment regimen, indications for surgery, evaluation of treatment efficacy and presentation of results vary in each report. It is scarcely possible to perform a randomized study with a group of untreated patients or to treat patients suitable for resection by other methods. A metaanalytic study using data published over almost 20 years would be questionable. Nevertheless we can draw some conclusions: the mean survival time of patients with extrahepatic tumours of the biliary tree treated with palliative implantation of metallic stents ranges from 4.6 to 14 months [14, 7, 24, 25, 26, 30, 37]. Combination with intraluminal and/or external beam radiotherapy can prolong it to 10-23 months (607 patients in 14 studies –Table 6), thus approaching the survival after radical resection of extrahepatic bile duct carcinoma (up to 23 months) [35]. Post- or pre-irradiation stenting seems essential for such prolongation.

Two factors of intraluminal irradiation account for these observations. First, the patency of the stent may be prolonged by delayed irradiated tumour ingrow into the stent lumen. This can postpone the stent occlusion with possible fatal complication. Second, if the tumour has a small diameter, its overall grow can be reduced, and the curative effect of irradiation can be considered. In our study, the survival time in Klatskin´s tumour grade III was longer than that of grade IV, but without statistical significance, probably due to a limited number of patients.

A number of studies of intraluminal brachytherapy combined with external beam radiotherapy and/or chemotherapy have been published recently, stressing the benefit of the combined modality treatment on survival [32, 45]. Veeze-Kuijpers et al. [45] compared the survival in patients receiving the combined modality therapy after surgery with that noted in nonresectable cases on intraluminal brachytherapy (median survival 15 month vs 8 month). Similarly, in study by Montemaggi et al. [32] the survival of patients with extrahepatic bile duct carcinoma on the combined modality regimen was longer than in patients treated by intraluminal brachytherapy alone. However the selection of patients receiving intraluminal brachytherapy alone was based on unfavourable findings (nonresectability, worse clinical status, larger tumour volume) in comparison with the selection for combined regimens. No data about postirradiation stenting were given. Alden [1] observed no differences in the survival of patients treated by external beam radiotherapy and intraluminal brachytherapy with or without palliative surgery. This study showed a positive correlation between the total dose of radiation and survival.

Complications: In our study there were no complications directly due to brachytherapy, which is in keeping with other studies using intraluminal radiation [32].

Conclusion: ILBT combined with stent implantation is a safe method, which appears to prolong survival in inoperable patients with Klatskin´s tumour and carcinoma of papilla Vateri compared with non-treated patients in previously published studies. In contrast no similar effect should be expected in patients with gallbladder carcinoma.

Table 6. Comparison of results of recently published studies using metallic stent implantation and radiotherapy in the treatment of biliary malignancies

Study	Tumour	No of patients	Radiation treatment (No of pts)	Stent (No of pts.)	Survival median (months)	Survival 1,2,3 years
Vallis KA et al 1996[44]	Cholangiocarcinoma	38	ILBRT⁺ + EBRT (14) / ILBRT⁺(4) / EBRT (20)	N.D.	15	N.D.
Eschelman DJ et al [10]	Cholangiocarcinoma	11	ILBT⁺	Gianturco	19.5*	N.D.
	Secondary tumours	11			5.3*	
Lee B et al. 1997 [26]	Cholangiocarcinoma	50	(8)	N.D.	8	25%, ?, ?
	Pancreatic ca	17	0		N.D.	N.D.
	Gallbladder ca	6	0		6.5	N.D.
Kamada T et al. 1996 [19]	Extrahepatic bile duct ca	103	ILBRT⁺+ EBRT	Metallic	14,9	55%,?,18%
				0	9,3	
Tsujino K. et al 1995 [42]	Extrahepatic bile duct ca	27	ILBRT⁺⁺ + EBRT	Surgical or PT	13	52%, 10%,?
Leug JT et al 1997 [28]	Extrahepatic bile duct ca	11	ILBRT⁺	(14)	12.5	47%,?,?
		4	ILBRT⁺⁺			
Leung J et al 1996 [27]	Cholangiocarcinoma	16	ILBRT⁺	(14)	23	61%,?,?
Fritz P et al 1994 [13]	Cholangiocarcinoma	30	ILBRT⁺ + EBRT	16 stent, other PTD	10	34%,18%,8%
Nunnerley HB et al, 1990 [34]	Cholangiocarcinoma	30	ILBRT⁺	N.D.	16.8*	N.D
Kuvshinoff BW et al, 1995 [22]	Hilar cholangiocarcinoma	9	ILBRT⁺ + EBRT	11 stent, 1 "T"-tube	14.5	N.D
		3	ILBRT⁺			
Mahe M et al, 1991 [29]	Klatskin´s tumour	20	ILBRT (8) ILBRT + EBRT (17) EBRT (25)	Surgical, PTD	12	55%,28%,15%
	Middle third tumour	23				

Table 6. (Continued)

Study	Tumour	No of patients	Radiation treatment (No of pts)	Stent (No of pts.)	Survival median (months)	Survival 1,2,3 years
	Distal, diffuse tumor	8				
Tana S et al, 1995 [41]	Extrahepatic cholangi-ocarcinoma	11	ILBRT[+] +EBRT	0	16.5*.	N.D
Alden ME et al, 1994 [1]	Extrahepatic cholangi-ocarcinoma	24	No RT	N.D.	5.5	N.D.
		13	ILBRT[?] + EBRT + CT		24	?,17%,?
		8	EBRT + CT		13.5	?,30%,?
		3	ILBRT		6	N.D.
Montemaggi P et al, 1996 [32]	Extrahepatic cholangi-ocarcinoma	18	ILBRT[?]+EBRT+ CT	4 PTD, 27 ERCP, no details	14	?,20%,?
Morganti AG et al [33]	Klatskin´s tumour	11	++ILBRT+EBRT+ CT	ERCP, no details	13	65%,33 %,? (5-year:14%)
	Gallbladder ca	1				
	Common bile duct ca	8				
Takamura A et al [40]	Klatskin´s tumour	75	++ILBRT+EBRT	PTD, different stents	11.9	49%,15 %, 10%
	Common bile duct ca	18				

*mean   ILBRT-Itraluminal brachytherapy, EBRT-External beam radiotherapy,
[+] Ir 192 HDR   CT- Chemotherapy, PT(D)- Percutaneous (drainage)
[++] Ir 192 LDR   Ca: Carcinoma
N.D. not determined   ? not known

References

[1] Alden, ME; Mohiuddin, M. The impact of radiation dose in combined external beam and intraluminal Ir-192 brachytherapy for bile duct cancer. *IntJRadiatOncolBiolPhys.*, 1994, 28, 945-951.

[2] Andersen, JR; Sorensen, SM; Kruse, A; Rokkjaer, M; Matzen, P. Randomized trial of endoprothesis vs. operative bypass. *Gut*, 1989, 30, 1132-1135.

[3] Bismuth, H; Castaing, D; Traynor, O. Resection or palliation: Priority of surgery in the treatment of hilar cancer. *WorldJSurg*, 1988, 12, 39-47.

[4] Cameron, Jl; Pitt, HA; Zinner, MJ; Kaufman, SL; Coleman, J. Management of proximal cholangio-carcinomas by surgical resection and radiotherapy. *AmJSurg*, 1990, 159, 91-98.

[5] Classen, M; Hagen,müller F. Endoprosthesis and local irradiation in the treatment of biliary malignancies. *Endoscopy*, 1987, 19, 25-30.

[6] Conroy, RM; Shahbazian, AA; Edwards, KC; et al: A new method for treating carcinomatous biliary obstruction with intracatheter radium. *Cancer*, 1982, 49, 1321-1327.

[7]   Coons, H. Metallic stents for the treatment of biliary obstruction: a report of 100 cases. *Cardiovasc Intervent Radiol*, 1992, 15, 367-374.

[8]   Dick, BW; Gordon, RL; LaBerge, JM; et al: Percutaneous transhepatic placement of biliary endoprostheses: Results in 100 consecutive patients. *J Vasc Interv Radiol*, 1990, 1, 97-100.

[9]   Dobelbower, RR; Merrick, HW; Ahuja, RK; Skeel, RT. 125I interstitial implant, precision high-dose external beam therapy, and 5-FU for unresectable adenocarcinoma and of pancreas and extrahepatic biliary tree. *Cancer*, 1986, 58, 2185-2195.

[10]   Eschelman, DJ; Shapiro, MJ; Bonn, J; et al: Malignant biliary duct obstruction: Long-term experience with Gianturco stents and combined-modality radiation therapy. *Radiology*, 1996, Sep, 200(3), 717-724.

[11]   Falkson, G; MacIntyre, JM; Moertel, CG. Eastern Cooperative Oncology Group experience with chemotherapy for inoperable gallbladder and bile duct cancer. *Cancer*, 1984, 54, 965-969.

[12]   Fletcher, MS; Brinkley, D; Dawson, JL; Nunnerley, H; Wiliams, R. Treatment of hilar carcinoma by bile drainage combined with internal radiotherapy using 192Iridium wire. *BrJSurg*, 1983, 70, 733-735.

[13]   Fritz, P; Brambs, HJ; Schraube, P; et al: Combined external beam radiotherapy and intraluminal high dose ate brachytherapy in bile duct carcinomas. *Int J Radiation Biol Phys.*, 1994, 29, 855-861.

[14]   Gillams, A; Dick, R; Dooley, JS; at al: Self-expandable stainless steel braided endoprosthesis for biliary strictures. *Radiology*, 1990, 174, 137-140.

[15]   González, DG; Gerard, JP; Maners, AW; De La Lande-Guyaux, B; Van Dijk-Milatz, A; Meerwaldt, JH; Bosset, JF; Van Dijk, JDP. Results of radiation therapy in carcinoma of the proximal bile duct (Klatskin tumour). *SemLiverDis.*, 1990, 10, 131-141.

[16]   Hishikawa, Y; Shimada, T; Miura, T; Imayo, Y: Radiation therapy of carcinoma of the extrahepatic duct. *Radiology*, 1983, 146, 787-789.

[17]   Johnson, DW; Safai, C; Goffinet, DR. Malignant obstructive jaundice: Treatment with external beam and intracavitary radiotherapy. *IntJRadiatOncolBiolPhys.*, 1985, 11, 411-416.

[18]   Johnson, P. The clinical features and natural history of malignant liver tumors. *ClinGastroenterol*, 1987, 17-34.

[19]   Kamada, T; Saitou, H; Takamura, A; Nojima, T; Okushiba, SI. The role of radiotherapy in the management of extrahepatic bile duct cancer: An analysis of 145 consecutive patients treated with intraluminal and/or external beam radiotherapy. *IntJRadiatOncolBolPfys.*, 1996, Mar 1, 3(4), 767-774.

[20]   Karani, J; Fletcher, M; Brinkley, D; Dawson, JL; Williams, R; Nunnerly, H. Internal biliary drainage and local radiotherapy with Ir-192 wire in treatment of hilar cholangiocarcinoma. *ClinRadiol*, 1985, 36, 603-606.

[21]   Klatskin, G. Adenocarcinoma of the hepatic duct at its bifurcation within the porta hepatis. An unusual tumor with distinctive clinical and pathological features. *AmJMed*, 1965, 38, 241-256.

[22]   Kuvshinoff, BW; Armstrong, JG; Fong, Y; et al: Palliation of irresectable hilar cholangiocarcinoma with biliary drainage and radiotherapy. *BrJSurg*, 1995, 82, 1522-1525.

[23] Lai, ECS; Tompkins, RK; Roslyn, JJ; Mann, LL. Proximal bile duct cancer: Quality of survival. *Ann Surg*, 1987, 205, 111-118.

[24] Lameris, JS; Stocker, J; Nijs, HGT; et al: Malignant biliary obstruction: Percutaneous use of self-expandable stents. *Radiology*, 1991, 179, 703-707.

[25] Lammer, J; Klein, GE; Kleinert, R; et al: Obstructive jaundice: Use of expandable metal endoprosthesis for biliary drainage. *Radiology*, 1990, 177, 789-792.

[26] Lee, BH; Choe, DH; Lee, JH; Kim, KH; Chin, SY. Metallic stents in malignant biliary obstruction: Prospective long-term clinical results. *AmJRoentgenol*, 1997, Mar, 168(3), 741-745.

[27] Leung, J; Guiney, M; Das, R. Intraluminal brachytherapy in bile duct carcinomas. *Aust N Z J Surg.*, 1996, 66, 74-77.

[28] Leung, JT; Kuan, R; et al: Intraluminal brachytherapy in the treatment of bile duct carcinomas. *AustralasRadiol*, 1997, 41, 151-154.

[29] Mahe, M; Romestaing, P; Talon, B; et al: Radiation therapy in extraheptic bile duct carcinoma. *RadiotherOncol*, 1991, 21, 121-127.

[30] Mathieson, JR; McLoughlin, RF; Cooperberg, PL; et al: Malignant obstruction of the common bile duct: Long-term results of Gianturco-Rösch metal stents used as initial treatment. *Radiology*, 1994, 192, 663-667.

[31] Meyers, WC; Scott Jones, R. Internal radiation for bile duct cancer. *World J Surg.*, 1988, 12, 99-104.

[32] Montemaggi, P; Morganti, AG; Dobelbower, RR; et al: Role of intraluminal brachytherapy in extrahepatic bile duct and pancreatic cancers: Is it just for palliation? *Radiology*, 1996, 199, 861-866.

[33] Morganti, AG; Trodella, L; Valentini, V; Montemaggi, P; Costamagna, G; et al: Combined modality treatment in unresectable extrahepatic biliary carcinoma. *Int Radiation Oncology Biol Phys.*, 2000, 46, 913-919.

[34] Nunnerley, HB; Karani, JB. Interventional radiology of the biliary tract. Intraductal radiation. *RadiolClinNorthAm*, 1990, 28, 1237-1240.

[35] Reding, R; Buard, JJ; Lebeau, G; Launois, B. Surgical management of 552 carcinomas of the extrahepatic bile ducts (gallbladder and periampullary tumor excluded): Result of the French Surgical Association Survey. *AnnSurg.*, 1990, 213, 236-241.

[36] Rossi, P; Bezzi, M; Rossi, M; et al: Metallic stents in malignant biliary obstruction: Results of a multicenter European study of 240 patients. *J Vasc Interv Radiol*, 1994, 5, 279-285.

[37] Salomonowitz, EK; Adam, A; Antonucci, F; Stuckmann, G; Zolikoffer, CL. Malignant biliary obstruction: Treatment with selfexpandable stainless steel endoprosthesis. *CardiovascInteventRadiol*, 1992, 15, 351-355.

[38] Siegel, JH; Lichtenstein, JL; Pullano, WE; Ramsey, WH; et al: Treatment of malignant biliary obstruction by endoscopic implantation of Iridium 192 using a new double lumen endoprosthesis. *Gastrointest Endosc*, 1988, 34, 301-306.

[39] Stain, SC; Baer, HU; Dennison, AR; Blumgart, LH. Current management of hilar cholangiocarcinoma. *SurgGynecolObstet*, 1992, 175, 579-588.

[40] Takamura, A; Saito, H; Kamada, T; Hiramatsu, K; Takeuchi, S; Hasegawa, M; Miyamoto, N. Intraluminal low-dose-rate 192Ir brachytherapy combined with external beam radiotherapy and biliary stenting for unresectable bile duct carcinoma. *Int Radiation Oncology Biol Phys.*, 2003, 57, 1357-1363.

[41] Tana, S; Di Russo, A; Cerrotta, A; et al: Transcutaneous radiotherapy combined with low dose intraluminal brachytherapy in the treatment of non-operable neoplastic stenoses of the bile ducts. *Radiol Med (Torino)*, 1995, 90, 124-128.

[42] Tsujino, K; Landry, JC; Smith, RG; et al: Definitive radiation therapy for extrahepatic bile duct carcinoma. *Radiology*, 1995, 196, 275-280.

[43] Valek, VA; Boudny, J. Interventional methods in the treatment of malignant conditions of the liver. *Cas Lek Cesk*, 2002, Aug 2, 141(15), 471-8.

[44] Vallis, KA; Benjamins, IS; Munro, AJ; et al: External beam and intraluminal radiotherapy for locally advanced bile duct cancer: Role and tolerability. *RadiotherOncol*, 1996, Oct, 41(1), 61-66.

[45] Veeze-Kuijpers, B; Meerwaldt, JH; Lameris, JS; Van Blankenstein, M; Van Putten, WLJ; Terpstra, OT. The role of radiotherapy in the treatment of bile duct carcinoma. *Int J Radiat Oncol Biol Phys.*, 1990, 18, 63-67.

[46] Venu, RP; Geenen, JE; Hogan, WJ; et al: Intraluminal radiation therapy for biliary tract malignancy – an endoscopic approach. *Gastrointest Endosc*, 1987, 33, 236-238.

[47] Washburn, WK; Lewis, WD; Jenkins, RL. Aggresive surgical resection for cholangiocarcinoma. *Arch Surg*, 1995, 130, 270-276.

Index

D

E

F

J

K

L

M

N

O

P

Q

R

U

V

W

X